Homoeopathic Acute Prescribing

A text for Practitioners, First Aid and Self-Help

Margaret Roy

The Scottish College of Homoeopathy

First published 2003. This edition published May 2005.

© Margaret Roy, The Scottish College of Homoeopathy

All rights reserved. No part of this publication may be reproduced, stored in a retrieval system or transmitted in any form or by any means – electronic, electrostatic, magnetic tape, mechanical, photocopying, recording or otherwise, without written permission from the publishers, nor be otherwise circulated in any form of binding or cover other than that in which it is published.

ISBN 0-9550415-0-3

Published by The Scottish College of Homoeopathy
17 Edinburgh Road, Biggar, Lanarkshire ML12 6AX

Typeset by Keystone Business Associates, Glasgow

Printed by Ritchie UK Ltd, Kilmarnock

Dedicated to

Bill and Peggy Bartlett

for a lifetime of kindness
and opening their hearts to others

Preface

I originally wrote this book for my introductory classes, hence it contains some basic introduction to Homoeopathy and some elementary Materia Medica.

As I continued I realised that, whilst we are very good at training students in constitutional prescribing, they are often less confident when it comes to acute prescribing. The rules are slightly different and the speed of action can be overwhelming to the new prescriber, so I have expanded the text to look thoroughly at treating acutes. The patient or self-help prescriber can only benefit from seeing their immediate problem in its larger context. Each lesson is organised to give a progressively deeper view of the Homoeopath at work. Hopefully this will enable patients to participate more fully in their treatment and understand some of our homoeopathic directions such as to wait, or even not to prescribe for the acute. I also hope it will enable the pharmacist, nurse, etc to look a little beyond the allopathic use of homeopathic remedies.

The Materia Medica in the book is based on having a 'First Aid' kit at home, so increasing its usefulness and encouraging a deeper appreciation of the remedies in hand.

With only a little knowledge, Homoeopathy is the safest and most efficient system of medicine known to us at this point in time. I hope this book will both encourage its use and increase the efficiency of that use.

Margaret Roy
May 2005

Contents

Introduction		9
LESSON 1	**First Aid with Homoeopathy I**	13
	First Aid Remedies, Homoeopathic Use in First Aid, Shock, Bleeding, Bruising, Wounds, Bites and Stings, Burns, How Homoeopaths look at symptoms, How remedies are made and stored, Provings, Dosage	
	Arnica, Hypericum, Ledum, Calendula, Cantharis	
LESSON 2	**First Aid with Homoeopathy II**	35
	First Aid Remedies II – Sprains and Strains, Healing Connective Tissue, The Law of Similars, More about Provings, Specifics, More about Dosage	
	Rhus toxicodendron, Ruta gravoleus	
LESSON 3	**Headaches**	49
	What are Headaches? Four Types of Headache – migraine, tension, sinus, bilious, Anatomy and Physiology, The Symptom Picture of a Headache, Maintaining Causes, Exciting Causes, Repertorising, Short Repertory of Headaches	
	Nux vomica, Pulsatilla, Bryonia	
LESSON 4	**Sore Throats**	63
	What is a Sore Throat? Philosophy, Individuality, Susceptibility, Precision, Clarity and Accuracy, Total Symptom Picture, Putting it all together, Remedies for Sore Throats, Throat Pain Repertory	
	Belladonna, Lachesis	
LESSON 5	**Earache**	79
	The Structure of the Ear, What is Earache? Acute Illness and the Level of the Disease Process, The Aggravation, Vitality, Remedies for Earache, Hering's Laws of Cure, Earache Repertory	
	Silicea, Hepar sulphuris, Mercurius	
LESSON 6	**Colds, Coughs and Flus – Winter Ailments**	91
	The Interaction of Three Factors in Disease, Winter Ailments – coughs, influenza, Remedies, Short Repertory of Colds and Coughs, Putting it all together	
	Gelsemium, Aconite	
LESSON 7	**The Digestive System**	107
	Digestive disturbance is a common occurrence, Maintaining Cause, Exciting Cause, Potency, Anatomy and Physiology, Travel Sickness, Food Poisoning, Colic, Dysentery, Remedies, Short Repertory of Digestive Symptoms, Putting it all together	
	Arsenicum album, Ipecacuanha, Ignatia, Colocynth	

LESSON 8   **Menstrual Problems**   125

The Nature and Role of Menstruation, So what can go wrong? Congestion, Exercise and Diet and the Maintaining Cause, Menstruation, Amenorrhoea, Dysmenorrhoea, Menopause, Causation, Concomitant Symptoms, Premenstrual Tension, Remedies, A Few Cases
Sepia, Cimicifuga

LESSON 9   **Rheumatism and Arthritis**   139

A Disease of Old Age? What is Rheumatism and Arthritis? A Homoeopathic Interpretation, The Acute Symptom Picture, Managing the Chronic Case, Some Remedies for Short Term Management, A Diet for Arthritis, Exercise, Remedies
Natrum muriaticum

LESSON 10   **Different Types of Acute Disease**   155

A Simple Acute, Vitality, Susceptibility, The Psoric Acute, The Acute Miasm, The Constitutional Case and Health, How is Vitality Changed? The Role and Types of Acutes in the Constitution Case, The Recurrent Acute, Episodic Acute, Acute of the Chronic, Where does epidemic, endemic, sporadic, contagious fit in? Potency and the Acute

Introduction

This book is about treating acutes. Amongst the assumptions in treating acutes is that they are simple, non-complex and can be dealt with at the self-help level. Whilst this is often the case, of course there is much more to the story. In this text I hope to give a clearer understanding of the acute process of disease.

In the homoeopathic approach to disease, any symptoms arise from within the organism as a defence response aimed at correcting disturbance. This gives us a very different attitude to the symptoms. We do not set about to cure symptoms but to understand why they are there and what they are doing. Symptoms are a pattern which indicates the state of the Vital Force – the complex matrix of life. In health there are no symptoms, so the presence of symptoms tells us there is an imbalance in the organism that we must understand in order to restore health. The natural state of the organism is health.

The Homoeopath has three causes of disease – exciting, maintaining and fundamental. These represent different types of disturbance of the vital energies, giving different meaning to the acute illness arising in each case and thus requiring a different approach to treatment.

The maintaining cause level is disharmony in the environment. Many symptoms, such as dullness of consciousness and loss of energy, arise from draining factors in our environment which are conditions inimical to life. Whilst medication might control these condition, it is obvious that action should be taken to improve the environment and/or personal habits.

First Aid can fit into the maintaining cause situation when an accident happens to an otherwise healthy person. Thus in First Aid situations restoration of health can be easy and simple with few underlying complications. The remedies are less individual in character because they are selected for similarity in the physiological process of defence and reparation. As we shall see in those lessons, there is still some individuality in the symptom picture as we each respond differently whatever the actual cause. Speed of resolution is affected by accurate choice of remedy. Differences arise from the underlying health of the organism that might cause it to act slower, for example, and therefore produce more suppuration in a wound than might otherwise be expected in a First Aid situation. Selection of potency after injury is usually the 30th centesimal that resonates on the *General* level where the defence mechanisms of the organism are uncompromised by underlying disease. Where the appearance of symptoms is slowed down by underlying dysfunction, or in the case of structural damage, a repeat dose of the 6th potency, will be discussed in the relevant section of text. External support as in a bandage or crutch becomes relevant and we should never ignore basic First Aid principles.

Detrimental environmental factors such as a stuffy atmosphere, overwhelming noise or too much sun might cause a headache. The most obvious treatment is to remove the patient or the maintaining cause then, through rest, allow the organism to restore itself. Samuel Hahnemann would call this pattern of disease pseudo-chronic – it will continue as long as the organism is exposed to the cause. However, these days we recognise that environmental poisons may be so insidious and exposure so prolonged that deeper adaptation is required to preserve the whole organism so the dysfunction created may take a bit longer to cure. Indeed the damaged or dysfunctioning organs may need help to recover. If we take the example of the tension headache, massage may be required before the muscles 'unlock' to release the tension. A homoeopathic remedy may speed up the relaxation and the excretion of toxins ingested or created during the organism's attempts to render the situation less harmful.

Sensitivity to such environmental factors varies from patient to patient until we become aware that the interaction is not just because of the volume or virulence of the maintaining cause. Where the patient is more sensitive, we may recognise an idiosyncrasy. Some may be more sensitive to heat whilst others produce an acute after exposure to cold. Now we are into the realms of the exciting cause that involves individual difference. This is what the Homoeopath would call the true acute.

When the acute arises from the exciting cause, the quality is different. The symptoms may arise as a group, or syndrome, that the patient recognises as typical of their reaction to the cause. The group of symptoms produced may not have a direct physiological relationship to the nature of the cause; for example, the sore limbs produced by the maintaining cause of over-exertion have a direct relationship to the over-exertion compared to the sore limbs produced in a flu after exposure to cold and damp, when the last is an exciting cause. In the last example it is the Vital Force that has been disturbed, not the Particular level. In the full symptom picture we will see a weariness and malaise accompanied by dullness of consciousness as the sore limbs develop 1 - 2 days after exposure. Other symptoms such as runny nose or headache will also develop to complete the symptom picture. In the maintaining cause situation the sore limbs will develop in direct proportion to the cause, differing only according to the vitality of the patient and there may not be other symptoms.

The acute arising from the exciting cause will vary according to the susceptibility of the Vital Force and its vitality which is now seen clearly related to the underlying health of the patient. An example here might be that, on exposure to cold, some patients will develop nothing because it is not their susceptibility, others may develop only a runny nose whilst less vital others might develop pneumonia or pleurisy. Yet others might develop earache because that is their individual weakness, or the old arthritis might start to trouble. Each of these examples relates to the ongoing chronic state of the Vital Force. Exciting causes are individual to each Vital Force in relation to the type of constitution.

The constitution is the fundamental cause. This is Hahnemann's theory of chronic disease. Why do we get ill in the first place? Why do we have weaknesses, or predispositions to ill health? Why do we develop symptoms as we get older, the diseases of old age? If you look at your family's health, in comparison to others, there are consistent patterns of disease. We have heart problems in my family. Is it true your family has nervous disorders? We get ill acutely according to the nature of the underlying weaknesses that have specific triggers or exciting causes.

To the Homoeopath the relationship between acute illness and the constitution is very important. Acute illness is thrown out by the Vital Force to restore harmony. More usually the constitution is silent but gradually breaks down as we get older. The constitutional pattern is a point of balance reached to accommodate chronic weakness but it is not 100% health. The compromise involves a point of gravity somewhat off centre. As we age, with the stresses of life, wear and tear, parts are eroded to produce the symptoms of old age. When there is sufficient extra energy the Vital Force will attempt to find a better point of balance but to do this it throws out an acute symptom picture. This is the point at which the Homoeopath can go grey-haired with exasperation as the patient reaches for the liniment, etc to suppress the symptom and the activity of the Vital Force. These acutes are very precious to the Homoeopath because the Vital Force is active and open to cure. They must be treated in such a way as to increase the movement outwards of the symptoms to lower the burden of imbalance (or toxicity). Indeed I would argue that this type of acute should never be treated except in relationship to the underlying fundamental chronic disease, especially when it is an acute miasm. An acute miasm is a childhood disease such as measles or chicken-pox that can so alter the economy of the Vital Force as to allow the child to overcome part at least of its inherited predispositions or weaknesses.

The Homoeopath can get into much trouble with orthodoxy in this approach to the acute. It must be remembered that the acute is not good in itself but only in its ability to create greater health. Indeed the acute according to Hahnemann was capable of either complete resolution or of killing the patient! Where there was not enough energy to deal with the acute the third option was, and is, to allow a deeper adaptation, slowing down reactivity but creating a disharmony in deeper tissue or structures. As we progress through life and the Vital Force has to respond to illness, you will note in many patients that illness becomes more and more serious. To follow one constitutional pattern, the pseudo-psoric miasm will produce tonsillitis in the child, acne and dysmenorrhoea in the teens, moving on to flus and bronchitis in the adult, then become more serious flus, bronchitis or even pneumonia, if not rheumatism, in old age. In treating these homoeopathically, the aim is not just to resolve the illness but to increase further the vitality of the patient. Indeed the raised vitality will reverse the process out of the respiratory system into the glandular. When we really hit the jackpot, as we can do in treating children, the energy released may give rise to a very violent acute. When this happens, it is necessary to understand the whole process of disease and to follow carefully Hering's Laws of Cure to determine the symptoms are flowing in a curative direction. Intervention may be required to keep the patient safe but hopefully this will be prescribed skilfully enough to enable the Vital Force to continue to lessen the chronic level of disturbance.

There are many types of acutes. Hahnemann speaks of four types – *epidemic, endemic, sporadic* and *contagious*. Each of these indicates a different relationship between Vitality, Predisposition and Exciting Cause. **Sporadic** illness picks out those that are susceptible, or of similar constitutional weakness or predisposition. An example might be a cold snap in March that brings a nasty cold. Of course weakened older people will be more susceptible because they have less vitality and here the cold snap might be seen as a maintaining cause! However, if you look at the sick population you will start to see the similarity of cold dry weather combined with weakness in the respiratory system. The *epidemic* is similar but wider spread, yet even here the population affected is much less than 100%. Indeed 20% will be an extraordinarily high figure. What does this group have in common? In flu epidemics the population may share the underlying constitutional weakness in the respiratory system and susceptibility to cold wet weather but this is not enough. The exciting cause is more virulent. Plus, if you look closely, there will also be lowered vitality. So the Homoeopath says that three factors are needed before an acute illness is produced – the **Predisposition**, the **Exciting Cause** and the ***lowered Vitality***. To improve vitality we look to environmental factors especially good food, water and air but also exercise and sleep, the five pillars of health. We tackle the predisposition by treating the patient constitutionally to raise levels of health – this is the only true preventative medicine. *Endemic* disease is related to an obnoxious environment inimical to life that eventually wears down the Vitality. It is akin to the maintaining cause.

Contagious disease is not the same as infection by micro-organisms. To understand this we must go deeper into the functioning of the Vital Force and of Homoeopathy. To those in the know it is the field theory of quantum physics – all similar substances will resonate. So the remedy works by resonating with a state of the Vital Force. But the remedy is a pattern of activity and the Vital Force is an energy so something changes or a process is initiated. When we hear our name or a catchy tune, or someone next to us starts to scratch or laugh or wink knowingly, we react. The child learns very early to mimic the adults, but it is more than that – it is picking up human characteristics as if it is in its very nature; of course that is it, nature. Through resonance our nature is awakened. Thus in disease, we do not all pick up the contagion, but if its nature is similar to ours, then we are more likely to. And note, in Homoeopathy, it is similarity not sameness that is the key to interaction! The same note will increase the volume; the resonant note will create a harmony.

There is another type of acute that it may be important to know about at this point. When health has degenerated, the organism throws off acutes more readily. The lesser the vitality, the more these are produced not from the exciting cause but from more flimsy exposure such as to a modality. These people may be very ill chronically so the acute is called the *acute of the chronic*. The point of balance is so precarious that it is very easily upset. An example might be a patient who develops 'bronchitis' as soon as he leaves his heated room and goes to the door where he is exposed to fresh air. Some symptoms are ongoing – his chest has been full of mucus for the last few years, he is breathless on the least exertion, he is easily chilled or tired out – but what he calls bronchitis is the appearance of a racking cough, expectoration rising and a slight temperature giving much greater discomfort. Certainly these are the symptoms of bronchitis, but notice the symptoms have not moved very far. Indeed in treating such a case it is very important to realise how little vitality the patient has and how slowly we must proceed with treatment … or else he will 'cough up his lungs'! At this level the body is overloaded with the products of disease and we must move slowly so it has time to excrete. Indeed treatment at first may be simply to increase the flow. Where a weakened constitution produces an acute, it needs skilful management to use that acute to improve vitality and thus health. The Homoeopath's skill includes the selection of an appropriate potency.

I will go into types of acute in more detail in lesson 10. In the text that follows, I hope to present material that will enable the student to explore the difference between the acute arising from the maintaining and exciting cause, and to relate acute treatment to the fundamental cause. The questions arising should help the patient in self-help to a deeper understanding of what they can help and what might be better dealt with by an experienced practitioner. Hopefully, it will help the patient to a deeper understanding of their health and therefore more informed participation in their homoeopathic treatment.

LESSON 1   First Aid with Homoeopathy I

First Aid Remedies

    Aims: To find out how to use homoeopathic remedies in a first aid situation.
                   To learn more about the remedies *Arnica, Hypericum, Ledum, Calendula, Cantharis*.
                   To begin the study of symptoms, especially to learn what is a full symptom – Time, Location, Sensation and Modality.
                   To find out how homoeopathic remedies are made, stored and tested.

New key words and concepts used in this lesson:

symptom	aetiology	Individuality
modality	keynote	symptom picture
proving	characteristic symptom	indicating symptom
Vital Force	Strange, Rare and Peculiar symptom	aggravation
constitutional remedy	Mental and Emotional symptom	amelioration
Total Symptom Picture	Particulars	Law of Similars

Homoeopathic Use in First Aid

A First Aid situation is when assistance is required to sustain life and/or prevent further damage to health in the absence of expert medical assistance – it is not a substitute for expert assistance.

For those of you who have not already done so, it is recommended strongly that you undertake a course in First Aid through St. Andrew's or St. John's Ambulance Association or The Red Cross. They will teach the order of assistance as Breathing, then Bleeding with special attention needed to Cardiac Failure, Unconsciousness and Spinal Injury using cardiac massage, artificial respiration, and how to support and contain injuries.

The use of Homoeopathy in First Aid is of enormous importance because of its effect on shock, bleeding and infection. It speeds up healing to a third of the normal time.

    Note: Because it is medicine, you must have permission from the patient before administering a homoeopathic remedy even in First Aid.

SHOCK

Shock may be emotional or physical. Bad news may hit us like a blow and we may respond as if it were a blow, taking time to recover from it. Our spirits may sink. We are overwhelmed so we cannot function normally. In this state the organism is deeply disturbed so healing time is needed – the Homoeopath would say the **Vital Force** is disturbed. Homoeopathy can speed up the healing time and recovery of the Vital Force. This is important because it is often shock that does the damage in accidents and it is shock that prevents efficiency of the healing. Thus there are three remedies to keep in your first aid box:

    Aconite   is the remedy used when we are frightened or experience 'shock' or trauma. Its action is upon the *fight or flight* mechanism – the patient is paralysed with fear. In extreme cases the patient may be struck dumb, or the offending limb may be paralysed literally. They *freeze*. It is said you can see the fear in the face of the *Aconite* patient. They are pale, may break out into a cold sweat, may wet themselves or suffer loose bowels, especially if it is a child. In severe cases the pupils may contract to pin pricks. Later on, they will be restless in sleep or even have nightmares. You could use *Aconite* after a child fell off a wall or off a bike. The fright is the main problem.

Ignatia is a common remedy for emotional shock where the patient is scattered (shattered in today's parlance.) They cannot settle to anything – cannot eat, sleep, think only of the subject matter and go over and over it in their mind. Often they will sigh. Sometimes there is a lump in their throat so they cannot swallow. It is a useful remedy to take before going to the dentist if you are afraid you will choke on all the saliva produced just by thinking of what might happen to you.

Arnica This a remedy for physical shock. Its proving symptom *as if hit by a blunt instrument* might often be referred to today in the words '*as if run over by a bus*'. It may occur in many different situations from physical blows after accidents, or even after viewing an accident. As in *Aconite* the patient may dream of the incident. Usually they will dismiss help or concern saying there is nothing wrong but their distance from normal functioning tells you there is something wrong. In severe situations this is the remedy of physical shock, especially after blood loss where the organism has to preserve life by drawing the blood from the extremities to the vital organs in the chest and abdomen. This gives the typical *shock syndrome* picture of pallor, cold sweat and weak thready pulse. We distinguish *Arnica* from *Aconite* in the mental reaction. One is anxious and frightened; the other says nothing is wrong and turns away. The pulse of *Aconite* is not weak but bounding.

> **PRACTICE POINT**
>
> A cup of tea or a warm blanket may console a shocked person and bring them back into contact physically and emotionally with the human race, but do not give anything internal if the patient is to be removed to hospital because of more serious injury – they may require an anaesthetic; do not overheat where there is risk of increasing bleeding, especially internally.
>
> Potency we will come back to. In shock you need to give at least a 30th potency but, depending on the severity, you might need a higher dose. Homoeopathy works best if you can give just one dose so it is good to think carefully about the potency you choose to do the job.

BLEEDING

Almost any homoeopathic remedy will stop bleeding if it is correctly indicated for the patient. There are specific remedies for certain types of bleeding, *Ipecacuanha* for arterial bleeding, *Phosphorus* for stringy nosebleeds, *Carbo Vegetalis* for slow oozing from small wounds. There is also in Homoeopathy the strange phenomenon of the *constitutional remedy.* There is nothing like it in orthodox medicine. How could there be one remedy that healed almost anything in the person for whom it is indicated? The legendary panacea! In Homoeopathy we treat the patient, not the part, because we accept that it is the Vital Force that is disturbed – that which maintains the integrity of the whole so that every symptom is part of a **Total Symptom Picture**. A constitutional remedy treats the whole so has an enormous range of action.

How do we select a remedy homoeopathically? We look for that which is individual or unique. Above we have the example of a **Mental and Emotional symptom** that distinguishes between two similar remedies. One is very frightened whilst the other pushes away any help. Both *Aconite* and *Arnica* may be effective in bleeding. The pulse is different where there is great disorder of circulation but more commonly it is the Mental and Emotional symptoms that makes the remedies entirely different.

Each remedy is unique in its characteristics, its field of action. When we look at symptoms homoeopathically, we look at aspects of **Time (Aetiology)**, **Location**, **Sensation** and **Modality**. It is this uniqueness that I will be drawing your attention to throughout this work. It is on this basis that we select remedies.

In Bleeding, re Location, we may choose a remedy such as *Aesculus* or *Phosphorus* for bleeding piles but we would look at *Phosphorus* or *Aconite* for nasal bleeding. *Bryonia* may be the indicated remedy if the bleeding were to take place at period Time, especially if the nasal bleeding came instead of the menses. Wherever the bleeding occurs we would think of *Phosphorus* if the bleeding were stringy, *Lachesis* if it were black, especially if clotted. *Phosphorus* blood is bright red.

Homoeopathy looks at detail to find that which is **Strange, Rare and Peculiar** or unique and **Individual** to this particular patient. How else could we describe bleeding? Well, sometimes it oozes or spurts. If it spurts, it may be arterial bleeding. This is where the First Aid course is essential to tell you how to use pressure and tourniquets to stop bleeding. The homoeopathic remedy *Ipecacuanha* has the characteristic of spurting bleeding so may stop the bleeding suddenly and spasmodically in arterial bleeding or in uterine haemorrhage especially after childbirth. It is quite startling to see bleeding being turned off like a tap but the First Aid course will teach that the next action is rest to allow the clot to form. The clot takes time to form so this advice is equally true in homoeopathic practice. Where bleeding oozes, two remedies come to mind – *China* and *Carbo Vegetalis*. The latter applies in venous types with poor circulation so the blood is often bluish. *Lachesis* and *Ledum* share the same features as *Carbo Vegetalis,* i.e. oozing bluish blood. To tell the difference you would need to go much deeper into the Total Symptom Picture to find out how this individual type is put together. It is a bit too simple to say that *Carbo Vegetalis* is dull and slow, *Ledum* is rheumatic and gouty, i.e. irritable, whilst *Lachesis* is negative in a bitchy, vindictive way or shy like a snake in the grass (the remedy comes from the venom of the Bushmaster snake).

PRACTICE POINT

Clean the wound with clean cotton, stroking away from the wound so as not to spread dirt and germs. It would be even better if your cotton were dipped in *Calendula* solution (see the table on page 29).

You may have to connect and tape the edges together or seek out help to stitch the ends of a wound. *Hypericum 30*, single dose, may help to close the wound and promote healing.

You may need to use pressure to promote the clotting mechanism or even a tourniquet. Back to that First Aid course!

BRUISING

This is a special type of bleeding that does not reach the surface. It is interstitial bleeding, between the cells, under the skin, giving rise to blue-black patches. By its nature it is usually caused by a blow *like a blunt instrument* – the signature tune of *Arnica*! Indeed *Arnica* is one of the major remedies in bleeding and bruising. It affects the clotting factor in the blood, creating a clot or dissolving one! This illustrates another major difference between a homoeopathic and a chemical medicine. A homoeopathic remedy has been tested until we know both of its actions. Any medicine by its nature has the ability to affect health. The Homoeopath states that a remedy has two actions, the first being opposite to the second. A homoeopathic remedy works because it can produce the same picture that is already present but the homoeopathic process can change this to its opposite, so curing. This is why we use the minimum dose to create change. More of this later.

If anyone was to take *Arnica* after a blow then the bruising may not occur. If you take the remedy after the bruising has appeared it will disappear much faster than otherwise, often the next day depending on the severity of the bruise. This is very important in head injuries where much damage can arise in concussion by pressure on the brain caused through the swelling involved in bruising. *Arnica* taken after the injury can stop the bruising or clear it up much faster. It is one of the very few occasions when I would recommend routine prescription without waiting for the full symptom picture to develop.

Arnica can be used before operations or even childbirth to reduce complications from bleeding and bruising. Additional benefits in childbirth include prevention of complications to the baby whose head has been squeezed out of shape in the birth canal. It is not necessary to give a separate dose to the baby because it will get the remedy from Mum through her milk. The Mum benefits greatly from *Arnica* before childbirth because the volume of the blood is reduced at one stage when the uterus contracts back to size. *Arnica* prevents clotting – very rarely embolisms can be formed at this stage of the birth process but seldom if *Arnica* is used. *Arnica* is a major remedy in thrombosis when its opposite action is to dissolve the clot. Depending on the potency it can do this very very fast so preventing coronary thrombosis, cerebro-vascular accidents (strokes) and embolisms of all sorts – probably even DVT! Of course, this is the realm of expert Homoeopathy but, once you have had a stroke, there is a high percentage probability that another will occur so it may be useful for the sufferer to carry *Arnica* after advice on how to use it. Swelling, bruising and blood loss occurring after broken bones may benefit from *Arnica* where the shock to the body confirms its use.

Ledum is a remedy of bruising where circulation is more sluggish so the bruising is yellow-green and long lasting. Because the system is so slow we use a low 6th potency and repeat it a few times whereas we only use one 30th potency of the *Arnica*. We would only repeat the *Arnica* if we had an indicating symptom such as pain to tell us the body still needed more help to cure itself. More of this later.

Arnica

We have already said quite a bit about *Arnica* so it might be useful therefore to study it here as a remedy.

It is a remedy with a profound effect on heart and circulation including bleeding and clotting. Its core theme or essence is *to centre*. Such a theme will run through all the symptoms and actions of a homoeopathic remedy thus enabling us to identify it even in situations (Time) when we do not expect to see it indicated. This movement to centre makes *Arnica* a major First Aid remedy where the response of the organism to injury is often to go into shock. Energetically the attention draws inward cutting off from the outside to rebalance or *re-centre*. Our language expresses the experience as *being knocked for six*, *run over by a bus*, or simply that *we need time to get over it*. We have been knocked off centre. Something has happened that we must integrate. *Arnica* speeds the process hence it is often used to speed up recovery before an operation or for jet lag.

The Mental and Emotional symptom picture of *Arnica* is so clearly in this vein of centring that it helps us identify the remedy easily. After the accident or incident, the *Arnica* patient wants to be left alone. They will withdraw temporarily into themselves and if disturbed will say nothing is the matter. Sometimes they are not in touch with what is the matter. The withdrawal into self allows them to rebalance and centre, i.e. integrate the experience.

In physiological terms Shock is a very specific process in which homoeostatic balance changes the distribution of the blood drawing it from the extremities towards the centre where the vital organs are located. Pallor is the first indication, or symptom, of this process. Chill may accompany it because there is less blood at skin level to maintain temperature. Where there is severe blood loss the full process produces a thready pulse and cold sweat. *Arnica* protects the heart and aids the blood loss by preventing further bleeding. *It restores integrity to the whole* is the signature tune or keynote underlying its action.

It forms clots and dissolves clots as explained in 'Bruising' above. The clotting process creates a barrier between parts and between the outside and inside world maintaining the integrity of the organism.

Thus in Homoeopathy *Arnica* is one of the major remedies for bleeding. In particular it is used where connective tissue is involved – that is bone, muscle and tendons. Examples might be tooth extraction and broken bones. In both of these cases the integrity of the whole is compromised. Bones give structure and form to the human body; muscles and tendons allow movement that is a main feature of the animal world. Wherever these parts are affected we find the keynote *fear of being approached or even touched*. There is sensitivity or a bruised feeling because where bones are broken or teeth extracted there is damage to the surrounding muscles and tendons and frequently blood vessels are torn. It is this additional damage that causes much swelling and pain. *Arnica* restores the integrity so fast that bleeding and swelling are prevented or reduced.

Another keynote of *Arnica* demonstrating this concept of integrity of the whole and 'attack' from without is *prickling from without inwards*. This unusual symptom can be seen where bone injuries are still healing (i.e. after the major pains have gone) and in the erysipelas that may arise where *Arnica* lotion is applied to open skin.

Arnica lotion that is frequently applied to aid bruised muscles and tendons should not be used where the skin is broken as it causes a sore, prickling inflammation of the skin.

A major characteristic Sensation of *Arnica* is the bruised feelings *as if the body was beaten*. These occur commonly in muscles where there is a blow but they also occur where there is over-strain. The resulting situation gives us further understanding of how *Arnica* works. The *pains are worse on first movement and better if movement is continued*. The build-up of lactic acid gives the bruised feeling but also indicates sluggish flow possibly because of congestion. Movement takes away the congestion but it is agony at first and better as the flow is established. It should come as no surprise that *Arnica* Location is especially the big muscles of the back where greatest integrity is held in the upright posture of the human being. Arnica becomes an excellent remedy for lumbago or those back pains after moving furniture or digging the garden. And these bruised pains are found during influenza attacks! The keynote symptom is *everything on which he lies feels too hard so there is constant movement to find a soft spot on the bed*. There is congestion and lack of flow. *Arnica* is a useful remedy for some kinds of flu and fevers but usually where there is gastric disturbance accompanying as in typhoid fever and dysentery.

The digestive symptoms of *Arnica* are characterised by sulphurous smells. When they belch it *smells and tastes of rotten eggs*. The flatulence *smells of rotten eggs*. If you remember Granny's use of Sulphur to cleanse the system, it may come as no surprise that the *Arnica* patient frequently produces boils – little vents that expel excess debris. Where we look at *Arnica* as a deeper remedy of heart and circulation we will find rheumatism and gout with red throbbing swellings around the large joints and the fear of being approached or touched. One of the ways in which circulation is compromised is through incomplete removal of the production of cellular digestion. These irritate the locality in which they are deposited giving rise to inflammation and pain. When the constitution is run down bruised patches, *ecchymosis*, may appear on the skin particularly in the extremities. When the constitution is run down or in some types of congestive illness, the main Mental and Emotional symptom is *irritability*. You can picture the chap with boils being very irritable!

The poor effects of digestion are to be found in other characteristic symptoms. The *Arnica* patient has a *craving for alcohol*. The stupor this drug produces can be found in the *Arnica* flu or fever and also in the head injury where there is another keynote symptom – *although unconscious speaks and answers correctly but relapses immediately back into unconsciousness*. This symptom is so inexplicable that it is a Strange, Rare and Peculiar symptom leading us directly to *Arnica* as the indicated remedy.

Modalities often give us a clear indication of a remedy or help us to distinguish it from a similar remedy. From above you can see when the *Arnica* patient will be worse for touch. In general the condition of *Arnica* may appear after exposure to cold, wet conditions, e.g. their rheumatism and bruised sore muscles may appear then. The exciting cause (Time) of *Arnica* is after injury. Then they are worse for the first movement and better for continued movement. Parts may be better for heat and rubbing them but the patient on the whole is worse for heat and touch.

> **EXERCISE**
>
> Homoeopathy is not a list of symptoms. It may help your memory to build up pictures of patients in certain situations, e.g. after breaking a leg, with boils, after a head injury, after tooth extraction.
>
> Use the keynotes and aspects of Time, Location, Sensation and Modality.
>
> You will find some help on this at the end of this lesson.

WOUNDS

These are the most common incidents in First Aid but in Homoeopathy, where we look at what is most individual, wounds come in many different types needing different remedies.

Calendula is used for grazes. These are wounds in which the epithelial lining tissue (Location) is stripped off or grazed. Since sensory nerves are abundant under the skin such wounds may be very painful. *Calendula* has the keynote symptom *pain out of all proportion* (Sensation). It is a remedy that restores integrity to epithelial lining tissue such as skin. Where there is grit in a graze it will push it out from within if the tincture is applied on a dressing. This is important in the case of young children who do not understand this pain or why you are digging out the grit. With *Calendula* you do not need to dig! *Calendula* **heals so well that it should be avoided in deep wounds where it might seal over the epithelial lining enclosing anaerobic bacteria such as tetanus**. In these cases *Hypericum* is used.

Hypericum is a remedy for deep wounds. As we will see shortly, its main effect is on nerves that are found in the deeper dermal layer of the skin (Location). We say it is a remedy of punctured wounds because the danger in these deep wounds is tetanus which attacks nerves. *Hypericum* is one of our most powerful remedies which protects nerves. It can be used to heal nerves when a limb is severed. Where this has happened surgically, *Hypericum* is used for the pain that appears in phantom limbs, i.e. where the nerve endings have been severed (Time). The symptoms are pains that shoot upwards along the tract of the nerve (Sensation). At the finger tips (Location) which are rich in nerves there is redness, swelling and throbbing drawing along the tract of the nerve, or there may be numbness (Sensation), e.g. after hitting the thumb with a hammer (Time). We will see this same redness, swelling and throbbing where the puncture has been caused by an insect bite (Time). A Strange, Rare and Peculiar symptom of *Hypericum* is that the pain will start up again if the wound is touched (Modality). *Hypericum* is also a remedy of suppuration where dirt has got into deep tissue structures.

Ledum is a similar remedy to *Hypericum* in that it is also used for deep or punctured wounds because it is a remedy of tetanus. Here the similarity ends as *Ledum* is a remedy of very poor circulation – so there is lack of oxygen. The wound is *numb, blue and cold* and so badly affected by heat that it is said to be *better from cold* (Modality). Where there are tetanus bacilli the *edge of the wound will twitch* (Location and Sensation). This wound is very slow to heal because of poor circulation. Where there is bruising, the colouring will be green and yellow, not black and blue. The remedy is often given after *Arnica* or *Hypericum* where these are slow to take effect because of the weaker or slower constitution.

Staphisagria is used when the injury has cut right across the nerves and tissue unnaturally ignoring natural 'channels' and lines of stress (Location). This produces a severe nerve pain described as *stabbing* (Sensation). We use this remedy after cuts by knives or operations

(Time). As a constitutional remedy its main theme is *outrage* or *indignation*. In terms of the body that is exactly what a knife or stab wound is. Is it not interesting that the *stabbing* type of pain in the constitutional remedy is reflected in First Aid use? And just to help you remember its use, it is also the remedy of 'honeymoon cystitis' appearing after first penetration in sexual intercourse (Time). In First Aid we use the remedy for shock where it is caused by rape, burglary, muggings, or other crimes of violence (Time) which *penetrate* our usual calm existence and gnaw at us so we cannot forget. We are indignant, outraged and even violated.

Hepar sulphuris is a remedy we use for suppurating 'dirty wounds' which are often found in children and animals who go out and get dirty again after the injury! The *raised red swelling produces thick, yellow pus*. This is one of the few occasions you will hear me suggest repeating the homoeopathic remedy. The reason is simply that this situation has been allowed to go on and develop and needs a bit more time to reverse the process. So we pace ourselves with the energy of the Vital Force, slow down by lowering the potency and repeat the dose as needed (until the wound starts to clear). Of course it might have been more use in the first place to try and keep the wound hygienically clean.

BITES AND STINGS

These are a special type of wound. Since they are punctures breaching the barrier of the skin, the two main remedies are *Hypericum* and *Ledum*. Here the suppurative aspect of both remedies may come to the fore as a bite or sting introduces foreign substance. Thus, as in *Hepar sulphuris* above it may be necessary to lower and repeat the potency.

Here we see the efficiency of the immune system. Different people react differently to a mosquito bite. Some will swell with redness, some come out in lumps, some lumps are exceedingly itchy. We call this Individuality. What is unique or Strange, Rare and Peculiar in a symptom picture enables us to match the similar remedy more precisely.

> **PRACTICE POINT**
>
> Remove stings carefully. Scrape a bee sting off with a knife. Do not press or squeeze as that releases even more venom from the sac protruding from the wound. With nettle stings, etc pull out in the direction in which they lie. Afterwards bathe the bee sting in baking soda and the wasp sting in vinegar. Rub dock leaves on nettle stings or midge bites.

Hypericum As in punctured wounds, the bite symptoms will be recognised by the red, swelling and throbbing if the remedy is *Hypericum*. The Modality > *cold applications*[1] can be seen to be appropriate here to bring relief. If the incident is severe enough there may also be characteristic red streaks drawing away from the wound and along the path of the lymphatic vessels showing the activity of the lymph system, i.e. the presence of poison. These symptoms will be present whether the bite is from a bee or a cobra. If it is a cobra you will need to use a much higher potency because the poison will be much more virulent! Personally, although my faith in Homoeopathy is well tried in bee stings and I would administer the *Hypericum* and expect it to work, in the case of cobra bites I would also make a bee line for the anti-venom serum – although I might delay just long enough to see the first symptoms appear! In bee stings, even *HYPER 30* aborts the symptom picture within seconds of being administered in highly sensitive types.

---

[1] The symbol > or < appears often in homoeopathic texts. They mean *better for* and *worse for* respectively.

Ledum may not be blue, cold and numb after being bitten by an insect but you will notice the swelling and numbness (Sensation). The swelling will take a long time to clear up because circulation is so poor or the uptake of fluid in the tissues is affected. The Modality remains << Heat. This remedy may be of use in rattlesnake bites. Of course this is not the usual First Aid situation and again you will need a very high potency if you are not driving speedily to the hospital for anti-venom serum, but that type of bite well illustrates the action of *Ledum* and what we mean by slow circulation. The way in which the venom of viper snakes works is by slowing down the blood, indeed by congesting and congealing it so it can no longer circulate and that is how death occurs. *Ledum* counteracts this action by speeding up circulation so there is no time to coagulate thus.

Note: Bee stings respond to *Hypericum* whilst wasp stings respond to *Ledum*. Trust me, I have five bee hives in my garden, so get some practice in.

Hepar sulphuris recurs in this section because many bites are 'dirty'. Bites from horse fly produce suppurating wounds. Rats, rabbits, dogs and cats, or humans for that matter, may not be too fussy re anti-sepsis. The symptom should still be a slightly raised lesion, red with thick yellow pus and very sensitive to touch (Sensation and Modality).

Apis mellifica is produced from honey bees. It is used where the bite or sting resembles that of the honey bee, i.e. hot, swollen, bright red, *shiny* and *stinging*. The appearance and the Sensation are both keynotes of this remedy. The Modality is > *cold applications*.

Urtica urens is a useful remedy to remember where there is swelling especially as vesicles (blisters), often an 'allergic' reaction to formic acid as in ant bites.

Cantharis can be used for vesicles, as with *Urtica urens* above.

Rhus toxicodendron is invaluable in cream form to take away the itch from midge bites.

Hypercal cream, a mixture of *Hypericum* and *Calendula*, is useful for any bite that you are worried might turn septic or be subject to tetanus, and it has the advantage of relieving the pain so is ideal for any little mishaps with children.

BURNS

Burns come in different degrees of severity, from blisters that cover a very small area to third degree burns that have removed much of the covering skin. Remedies may differ according to how the burn has affected, its Individuality, or the main physiological effect produced.

> **PRACTICE POINT**
>
> Cold water is usually recommended for scalds to prevent further heat dissipation. For small areas, many Homoeopaths will tell you warm water is better and homoeopathic. You have to try this to believe me.
>
> Where the skin is broken, hygiene is very important to prevent sepsis. If very severe, the burnt clothes (which have been sterilised) are often left protecting the open wound until the patient is in hospital. This also prevents the delicate skin from being ripped off too.

Hypericum is commonly used for burns. The skin is red, fiery hot, swelling and throbbing – the same signature tune of *Hypericum* we saw in wounds. As in deep wounds, because it promotes granulation in the dermal area of the skin, its action may prevent sepsis that is a major cause of death in burns. To achieve this we cover the skin with a dressing soaked in *Hypericum* tincture to protect from outside interference. Where the burn is deep or covers a large area destroying much of the skin, the dressing is left in place for up to two weeks undisturbed except for further applications of *Hypericum* as needed – pain can be a good indicator of further doses although this can be controlled by *Hypericum 30* by mouth. These are applied to the dressing which is then covered by a second dressing that is removed as needed to apply the *Hypericum* tincture to the lower bandage. This procedure protects the growing skin beneath and usually prevents scarring. With today's dependency on a medical culture it may take courage to leave such a wound for two weeks but countless cases homoeopathically testify that after that period a new skin is formed.

Cantharis is the remedy used when fluid balance is disturbed. Loss of fluid is the second major cause of death from burns. *Cantharis* is used wherever soft tissue is burnt, e.g. mucus membrane inside the mouth (Location). When *Cantharis* is the indicated remedy homoeopathically, blisters are formed. I have experienced these disappearing before the patient has finished sucking the remedy. The pain may go as soon as the remedy is in their mouth! In more serious burns there is a great deal of fluid loss and even kidney failure due to lack of fluid. *Cantharis* is still the remedy but is now required in much higher potencies. Of course, this needs more expert prescription as in the deeper case of *Hypericum* above.

Urtica urens comes from the stinging nettle. Like *Cantharis* it is best used where there is fluid imbalance shown by blisters but it is one of the best remedies I know for sunburn with its red raw then dry, flaking and stinging (Sensation) symptom picture. It feels just like a nettle sting. It is a very useful remedy to know about because it grows so prolifically in so many countries. To make use of it, boil it in water for 20 minutes then add honey and apply it to the area.

Belladonna is one of the most invaluable remedies for sunstroke especially where the fever rises to give a very hot and full head (Sensation and Location). The fever can be seen in the redness of the face. The heat can be felt to radiate from the face. Delirium may ensue, especially in children.

Hypericum

This is a most useful remedy to keep in your First Aid box because of its profound effect on nerves. The most use in the home will be to protect the nerves from the tetanus bacilli. J. T. Kent, one of our greatest Homoeopaths, never used any homoeopathic remedy routinely except this one. Mind you 100 years ago there were more horses and their dung about!

Pain is the main indictor of *Hypericum*. Locally this is *throbbing* (Sensation) sometimes shooting up the tract of the nerve towards the centre of the nervous system. The most common parts affected are the fingertips that are rich in sentient nerves (Location). If hit by a hammer, or jammed in a door, these will produce the *numbness* of nerve involvement then the tip will *swell*, become *red* and *fiery* and throb intensely. Bunions and chilblains equally respond well to *Hypericum* with a similar symptom picture in similar location, extremities rich in nerves, i.e. toes. Another Location where injury demands *Hypericum* is to the tailbone after a fall (or even after childbirth where this is a common injury).

Hypericum is to be found indicated wherever nerves are affected. It is indicated in pain in phantom limbs after amputation and can be used to reconstitute the nerve connection where parts have been almost severed. The pain on this level will definitely have the Individuality of *shooting along the tract of the nerve towards the spine*. Any damage to spinal nerves may require *Hypericum*. A common injury to the spine is concussion when one mis-steps off a pavement. The spine is very sensitive to touch. In head injuries where *Hypericum* is indicated the head *feels numb* and there is a Strange, Rare and Peculiar symptom of *as if the feet will rise over the head on lying down*. The brain of course is full of nerves. Today, in its crude form as St. John's Wort, *Hypericum* is often used for depression. The Homoeopath will use it where depression arises after head injury.

The use of *Hypericum* in burns and toothache is based on its effect on nerves. In the first the nerves are damaged and intensely painful. In the second the nerves are attacked by decay. *Hypericum* is a remedy of suppuration, overcoming bacterial invasion. As said above, in burns, this prevents sepsis that is a major cause of death. The burnt person is extremely vulnerable because the protective layer of the skin is missing. Where the suppuration process is active in a *Hypericum* patient there are *red streaks* in towards the body and along the line of the lymphatic vessels.

Modalities – what would affect nerves? It should come as no surprise that the *Hypericum* patient is worse if touched or on pressure and better lying quietly.

Ledum

This is a constitutional remedy of worn down constitutional types who have abused their body, such as alcoholics. Notoriously it is a remedy of gout and ecchymosis (bruising) in the extremities through poor circulation. In the end it is a remedy of heart disease.

With this in mind we can understand where it comes in as a First Aid remedy when circulation has been slowed down as in some types of insect bite or sting, or for the bites of viper-type snakes. It suits old wounds that are not healing or slow to heal. Hence in bruising the coloration is *greeny-yellow* as in old bruises. It is invaluable where *tetanus is kept local* because of poor circulation. Then the area around the wound itself is *seen to twitch*.

Symptoms are local. The characteristic process of *Ledum* is *creeping so chills ascend from the feet* (Sensation and Location) in rheumatism. In the wound there is *coldness, blue coloration and numbness* (Sensation). The coldness and blue colour come from absence of blood. Movement that increases the flow of blood, especially heat, is an aggravation; so much so that the keynote is *cold > cold* (Sensation with Modality).

This poor circulation makes *Ledum* a very useful remedy in eye injury where the cause is a blow creating a bloodshot eye or black eye. The eyelid may even be seen to twitch.

The itching is more common under the skin in liver congestion but it may occur in First Aid where a bite continues to itch as it is slow to heal (Sensation).

Modalities – we have already explained why the *Ledum* patient is worse for motion and heat and better for cold.

> **EXERCISE**
>
> I wonder what your drawing skills are like? Can you draw two pictures to distinguish between these two remedies? Or maybe you could find and cut out a magazine picture so you have the stereotype firmly identified.

Calendula

This is such a small remedy in terms of its symptom picture but who has not heard of its use, indispensable in wounds? It creates aseptic conditions. Try putting a little mince in a *Calendula* solution – it should not rot!!! Asepsis means that no germs can live in its presence so the Homoeopath uses it especially to wash out wounds but also for mouthwashes, and I use it on planes as a barrier to infection.

It has a particular affinity (Location) for epithelial lining tissue such as skin. Like *Arnica* it acts to restore integrity, in this instance the covering function of skin. The typical wound will be a graze where the ragged edges are said to resemble the leaves of the plant. The keynote symptom *pain out of all proportion* (Sensation) makes it indispensable for children when they have those grazes that are full of grit. Do not bother picking out the grit piece by piece. Simply irrigate the wound with a 1:40 dilution of the mother tincture (often supplied ready made-up) then wait for the unique action of the remedy to push out the grit overnight. Because of the sensitivity to pain it has also been used as a dressing for bunions! And *Calendula* soap is not to be sniffed at for stopping those blackheads from becoming infected and then spots.

The sensitivity to pain should give you the idea of the type of person, i.e. a sensitive type who is *exhausted by the pain*. The same type is sensitive to cold, > *warmth*, and *low in spirits in cloudy weather* (Modalities). The plant is the Marigold that opens its bright orange flowers to the sun, and closes then when the sun goes down. You can see by this that it is a remedy for lowered vitality. Indeed its other main use in Homoeopathy is in cancer where it restores the integrity to epithelial lining tissue such as the surface of organs where carcinomas form. (J. H. Clarke has some interesting cases here.)

Cantharis

This remedy is derived from an iridescent Spanish fly that causes irritation or even blisters when touched. Thus it is used in burns that blister but in fact the remedy's affinity is for lining tissue that keeps moist, i.e. the lining of the inner tubes, especially the urinary system (Location). As such it is frequently indicated in acute cystitis. It is for these two conditions that we keep it in the First Aid box, usually in a 6th potency as a 30th potency would indicate something much more serious that would need expert help. Also, in a 30th potency, it will affect more deeply and another action of this remedy is to slough off lining tissue, hence its use to clean out the womb after miscarriage.

Its signature tune re symptoms is severe *itch that burns* (Sensation). This may be in piles or intestines. The parts may turn black but first we will see a *rawness* (Sensation) of the parts that the organism protects with stringy mucus. Any discharges may become *bloody and acrid* which you can apply also in sore throats, if the rest of the symptom picture agrees. The parts affected are < *touch* (Modality), as you would expect where there is irritation. *Eruptions burn when touched* (Sensation). When the symptom picture deepens irritation may become spasm (Sensation). This is where we get some of the Strange, Rare and Peculiar symptoms of *Cantharis*. The sore throat will go into spasm on drinking water, ultimately there will be *spasms at the thought of drinking water, or even sight of water*. In urinary problems there is spasm that stops the action of the bladder, *retention < drinking water*. Another keynote that appears in urinary problems is *constant urge to urinate but only a few drops produced*.

This last symptom can extend to the personality type who is *restless*, constantly on the go, *constantly attempting to do something but accomplishing nothing*. Here the irritation becomes dissatisfaction and contradiction [2]. They are touchy types but in the sense that ideas touch them leading to a frenzy so they may go into a rage and bite like *Belladonna*, not really common in a First Aid situation. You may not see the *singing of lewd songs* but you will recognise the *strong sexual desire*.

---

[2] Such mental and emotional symptoms are a bit more than Sensation. Likewise spasm, although a Sensation borders on dysfunction. And on this subject, you will notice that there is not much Time. Time is the point at which it all begins, that might be a Time Modality as in *Belladonna* < 3pm but more often it is the Exciting Cause – we will see this in the next few lessons.

Remedies can have an enormous scope of symptoms but it does not mean that the patient has to have **all** of the symptoms. There may be a progression into disturbance so the most notable keynotes are often not present in a case. Then the Homoeopath will look for the components of the Essence of the remedy. Here that will be the itch that burns, the aggravation to touch and the spasm that is sensitive to drinking water.

SUMMARY OF PHILOSOPHY LEARNED IN THIS LESSON

We talk of Homoeopathy as an **alternative**, or sometimes complete, **system of medicine**. Here is why.

The underlying philosophy is different from orthodox or Western medicine in that Homoeopathy treats the whole person – each and every symptom of a patient is gathered in the interview to form a **total symptom picture**. It is difficult to treat a symptom in isolation homoeopathically. Each symptom is studied as to where it fits into the whole picture. What pattern is formed? This is because Homoeopathy does not see the symptom as the disease or illness. Homoeopathy belongs to that school of philosophy called Vitalism which means we see the being held together by a force called the **Vital Force**. There is no difference chemically between a living and dead body but the dead body cannot maintain its integral wholeness – it disintegrates. Life itself is absent.

Like electricity or magnetism, we cannot see or smell the Vital Force. We know of it only by its effects – it produces **symptoms**, signs of discomfort outside the ordinary. Indeed the Vital Force maintains health but when it is working well we do not notice this. It is only when things go wrong that symptoms draw our attention that there is a problem. The Homoeopath studies the pattern of symptoms to find a remedy that has a similar **symptom picture**.

What we have learned so far about symptoms is that they have four aspects – Time, Location, Sensation and Modality. We could add a fifth – **Intensity**. A full symptom to the Homoeopath has all of these aspects giving a pattern of **Precision**, **Clarity** and **Accuracy** [3]. We may go into gruesome detail here when **taking the case** (finding the symptoms during the interview with the patient).

We mentioned **types of symptoms**. There are five types of symptoms homoeopathically –

- Strange, Rare and Peculiar
- Mental and Emotional
- General
- Particular
- Common

These give a hierarchy of importance. Strange, Rare and Peculiar symptoms are illogical and inexplicable. They are so unusual and **individual** that they point directly to one remedy or to a very small group of remedies so they can save us a lot of work. Mental and Emotional symptoms are very important in the **constitutional remedy** indicating what is most characteristic and individual about us. General symptoms correspond to metabolism as a whole and so include sleep, breathing, appetite, digestion, excretion, urination, menstruation, sex, sweat. Notice these terms refer to processes. The product of the process, or the apparatus (organ) allowing it, is a **Particular**. Particulars are the bits and pieces where the symptoms show particularly as pain.

Common symptoms are a bit tricky homoeopathically. They refer to the common patterns of symptoms that group together to give the doctor disease labels such as hepatitis, arthritis, asthma, typhoid. The Homoeopath rarely prescribes on them but they are very important in allowing us to separate out what is individual and unique.

In studying a symptom picture homoeopathically we are looking for what is **individual** and **unique**. J. T. Kent, one of our greatest Homoeopaths, says a **prescribing symptom** is something that makes us

---
[3] See George Vithoulkas in *The Science of Homoeopathy*

stop and hesitate [4]. What I have picked out in the text above and what you will see in the little books in some health stores are the special identifying symptoms of the remedy – the **individuality** that is its signature tune, or **Keynote**.

Homoeopathy has 2000+ remedies. Each is unique in character. At this level of study the Keynotes are invaluable in helping us to recognise a remedy.

SUMMARY OF PRACTICE POINTS SO FAR

1. Find what is most individual and unique in the case. Match these to the symptom picture of a remedy.

2. It is not enough to give a remedy. Convalescent time is needed to allow the healing process, e.g. in bleeding for the clot to form.

3. Hygiene cuts down on healing time. Use *Calendula* 0 diluted 1:40. Wet cotton wool and use strokes away from the wound.

4. In burns do not change the dressing ripping off the new skin. Soak the underdressing in *Hypericum* solution. This acts as a painkiller and is antiseptic. Use the top dressing to keep it all dry and clean.

5. Use *Hypericum 30* routinely for tetanus.

6. Use *Arnica 30* routinely for head injury – and get help.

7. To repeat the dose find an indicating symptom such as pain. That way you work *with* the Vital Force.

8. Use repeat doses in low potency when you expect physical draining and repair, or low vitality, to slow the process.

Remedies

How they are made

There are four sources of remedies – minerals, plants, animals and human disease tissue. The largest group is the plant group, although many remedies are minerals such as Sodium Chloride (*Natrum muriaticum*), Sulphuric Acid, Gold *(Aurum)*. Animal venoms form a very small group, snakes and spider venoms in the main, but also well known remedies such as Sepia derived from the ink bladder of the cuttlefish that squirts it to form a cloud in which it can hide. Human disease products have the special name of **nosodes**. They are a very small but most important group that removes the family disease diathesis (the inherited tendency to have heart or respiratory problems, etc).

Whatever their source, remedies are ultimately put into a solution to form the *mother tincture* from which all other potencies derive.

The mother tincture is diluted 1:10 on the **decimal scale**, 1:100 on the **centesimal scale** to form the first **potency**. A further dilution of 1:10 or 1:100 from the first potency will give rise to the second potency and so on. The strength of the potency is defined on the label, after the name of the remedy, by a number and either the letter **X** for decimal (**D** on the Continent of Europe) or **C** for centesimal.

Between each dilution the mixture is shaken violently in a jarring manner called **succussion**. Apart from the mother tincture and the final solution that use alcohol as a preservative, water is used as a

---

[4] See J. T.Kent in Lectures on *Homoeopathic Philosophy*

solvent. For almost two centuries Homoeopathy has been abused as no more than a placebo effect (or worse) because of this process of dilution and succussion. It is only with the arrival of quantum physics applied to biology that we have found that DNA contains memory through the properties of water which is imprinted with the nature of the original substance. After so many dilutions (Avogrado's number is 24**X**), it is said that no molecules of the original substance remain in the solution.

This process is called **potentisation**.

How to handle and store them

Most remedies are in pilule or tablet form although the form may be liquid, tincture. One drop only is added to 7 gm pills made of lactose or sucrose. This one drop contaminates the pills. Now, if we are talking of contamination and if one drop is sufficient then there is an inherent degree of fragility. Homoeopathic remedies are very sensitive to handling when the sweat off the hand can destroy the potency. Strong smells are taboo by their very nature – they are infinitesimal pieces of matter (not unlike homoeopathic remedies). Remedies are sensitive to heat and light so are stored in dark bottles away from direct heat and strong smells.

Provings

From where do these symptoms arise?

The story goes that Samuel Hahnemann was translating a book by William Cullen of Edinburgh University. In part he saw the use of quinine for malaria. Having been a doctor at the front in the Napoleonic Wars, Hahnemann knew quinine worked so he set out to find why. He took the medicine himself then developed the symptoms of malaria. He then understood that every medicine has two actions, the first being opposite to the second. If the first action is to produce the symptoms then the second action is to cure those same symptoms. Thus in Homoeopathy we seek a remedy that will produce the same symptoms the patient already has. This is the **Law of Similars**, like cures like. The remedy increases those symptoms, the *aggravation*, then follows the *amelioration*.

Once he had worked out this approach to therapeutics, all he had to do was to 'prove' the remedies by taking them then noting the patterns of symptoms produced and then cured. This process is the homoeopathic **proving**. From the proving we determine the symptom picture of a remedy – its field of action, or resonance, those symptoms it can cause and cure.

From Hahnemann's day, almost 200 years ago, Homoeopaths have collected symptom pictures in books called *materia medicas*. 200 years later we are still making good use of Hahnemann's work showing it is not arbitrary but repeatable phenomena, i.e. scientific.

Dosage

I expect you will be wondering about this. It is not an easy subject for the Homoeopath because we not talking of chemical doses. You could take a whole bottle of homoeopathic pills and not overdose. Indeed I have had several patients phone up in despair that their child has swallowed **all** their supplies of First Aid remedies. They come to no harm as long as the pills were swallowed in one sitting. I had one art student who tried to commit suicide by swallowing many of my bottles of pills. She could not understand hours later when nothing had happened. This is not how Homoeopathy works.

The Single Dose

We use one pill. When I first started to practise I could not believe that **one** pill could do much so I used to give a Collective Single Dose, CSD – three pills taken with three hours between each.. I was very surprised when I realised that **one** pill was more potent. How you ask?

Homoeopathy works on the laws of physics, not chemistry. It is energy we are handling and we have specially prepared the medicines of different energies, or potencies. Remember it is not the symptoms we are treating but the Vital Force which is an energy. How do you change the course of action of a river? You could stand there as it bore down on you. You would only affect that bit of water. Like the wind, that bit of water would flow past but the forces that kept the river or the wind flowing would still be unaffected. You need to get to causes. Where is the river or the wind coming from? Do you want to change it or just change its direction of flow? If the Vital Force creates the symptoms then it is the Vital Force we must change, but the Vital Force is an energy we know so little about. At least with the river we could have built a dam!

The Vital Force is intelligent. The remedy is information. How many times do I need to tell you how to do something? The information is passed with one pill, the single dose. The Vital Force can choose what it is going to do with the remedy. It has an order of priorities. It knows when something is wrong even before the symptoms appear. It will take from the remedy what it needs. If there is no resonance, the remedy will have no effect. The absolute safety of Homoeopathy is built around this premise. If there is no resonance, the remedy will have no effect.

The greatest difficulty to the beginner to Homoeopathy occurs when the voice, the remedy, is not loud enough for the Vital Force to hear. I suggest to students that they repeat the dose if nothing happens. Wait only 20 minutes in a case of headache. If nothing happened to stem bleeding within minutes of taking a homoeopathic remedy repeat the dose or find another remedy, fast. In First Aid where the organism is basically healthy the Vital Force should respond really fast. When you give a remedy only three things can happen:

1. The symptoms improve. Why give more medicine then?

2. The patient gets worse. Why give more of **that** medicine? If it is making the patient worse, do not repeat the medicine. Sometimes homoeopathically you get worse before you get better. This happens because symptoms are the process of expelling disorder so this process of expulsion may initially be speeded up. This is the best thing that can happen after a homoeopathic remedy and the last thing you should do is interfere with the healing process. **Note:** diarrhoea, vomit, catarrh are increased, **not bleeding** which is a vital process.

3. If nothing happens, you must ask why. Look at all the symptoms. Sometimes the patient is only looking at one symptom, or the change was too deep for us to see. Give another dose of the remedy, at an interval depending on how serious the condition. If you need to give yet another dose you must seriously review the remedy chosen or look to see if there is something much more important that the Vital Force has to attend to first. **Seek expert help here.**

Potency

The most common potency available is the sixth centesimal. Once you have just a little bit of knowledge, as after doing this course, you may use the thirtieth centesimal potency where the situation is more severe or you need to move the symptoms faster – but not with young children who are very sensitive. With a single dose of the thirtieth centesimal potency you will see very clear patterns of change.

It is possible to overdose slightly but if you follow the rules above you will not give a second or third dose. If you happen to give a second unneeded dose, the Vital Force will cure the problem then go on to produce other symptoms that we call **proving symptoms**. These should disappear harmlessly in a few hours or days depending on the speed of appearance.

Where the healing rate is slower, as in sprains and strains or festering wounds, you need to match the speed of cure by using a slower lower potency, the sixth centesimal. In these situations, as explained above, you will need to repeat the dose.

PRACTICE POINT

A useful indication as to the effect of a remedy is the length of the gap before relapse of symptoms.

The beginner in a self-help situation is not expected to get it absolutely correct, therefore it is probable that the symptoms will return – that is all right.

Study the symptoms. If cure is taking place, the gap between relapses should get shorter and the intensity should get less. If this happens after you give the second dose then it is all right to go ahead and repeat the medicine but if you need to repeat beyond three doses, get expert help – something is not quite right.

SUMMARY

PROBLEM	REMEDY	SYMPTOMS	DOSE
SHOCK	*ACONITE*	Paralysis – shock still. Cold seat, pale, bounding pulse. May pee themselves.	ONE 30th potency Repeat only as needed, i.e. after a nightmare or if anxiety returns.
	IGNATIA	Emotionally overwhelmed or scattered – restless, change subject, or cannot settle to anything, can't eat, can't sleep, can't concentrate. Lump in throat.	ONE 30~200~1M depending on blow. Repeat as emotion returns.
	ARNICA	As if hit by a blow – physical or M/E. Thoughts of it recur.	ONE 30th potency Repeat as symptoms recur.
		Physiological shock after injury. Cold extremities, cold sweat, thready pulse, pallor. Say to go away, nothing wrong.	ONE 6th potency and repeat if very weak. 30th potency if or as gets stronger.
WOUNDS	*CALENDULA*	Surface grazes. Much pain.	Tincture 1:40 to wash out wounds with cotton wool re sepsis.
	HYPERICUM	Deeper cuts or punctures. Sweating, redness, bleeding, sensitive to touch. Throbs and shots upwards.	ONE 30th potency Repeat with pain. Dress wound with tincture.
		Nerves affected. Injury to parts rich in nerves.	ONE 30th potency Repeat with pain.
	LEDUM	Deeper cuts and punctured wounds. Numb, cold, < heat. May twitch around the edges.	ONE 30th potency for tetanus if serious. Dress wound with Hypercal. Or REPEAT 6th potency every 3-4 hours.
	STAPHISAGRIA	Cut across nerve and tissue. Stabbing pain + shock with indignation and helplessness.	ONE 30th potency Repeat with pain or return of emotion. If emotion persists rise to 200th potency.
	HEPAR SULPHURIS	Suppurating wounds – boils, cuts, scratches, etc. Yellow pus, very sensitive around edges.	Repeat 6th potency 3-4 hours.
HEAD INJURY	*ARNICA*	From a blow, may feel bruised or sore.	ONE 30th potency Repeat as needed with pain.
		Consciousness is lost but returns as the patient is spoken to, then they drift off again.	ONE 30~200~1M depending on severity. Give nothing by mouth – pill only needs to touch tissue lining mouth. Get help.
	HYPERICUM	There is a numbness or a dizziness indicating nerve involvement.	ONE 30th potency Repeat as symptoms return.
		In severe cases there is a sensation as if the feet rose over the head.	ONE 200~1M potency Repeat as symptoms recur.

PROBLEM	REMEDY	SYMPTOMS	DOSE
TETANUS	*HYPERICUM*	Dog bite, cut from garden, etc. Red, swollen, throbbing. Red streaks extend upwards along the lymph vessels.	ONE 30~200~1M depending on severity.
	LEDUM	Old punctured wounds that are cold, bluish and twitch, especially when touched.	Repeat 6th potency every 3-6 hours.
BLEEDING	*ARNICA*	Bruising. Feels bruised and sore.	ONE 6th potency (child) 30th potency adult
		Pre-operation	ONE 30th potency 6-8 hours before. Repeat if needed afterwards for pain and bleeding.
	LEDUM	Bruising. Yellow-green, slow to arise and very slow to resolve.	Repeat 6th potency every 3-6 hours.
	ACONITE	Nosebleeds. Bright red blood, bounding pulse. Fear or anxiety.	ONE 30th potency Repeat as recurs.
	BRYONIA	Nosebleeds at time of menses.	ONE 30th potency Repeat if recurs.
	PHOSPHORUS	Nosebleeds – bright red, stringy blood.	ONE 30th potency Repeat as recurs.
		Piles bleeding – bright red possibly with some mucus.	ONE 30th potency Repeat as recurs.
	AESCULUS	Bleeding piles in congestive type.	Repeat 6th potency every 3-6 hours.
	IPECACUANHA	Bright red in spurts. May have nausea and faintness.	ONE 6-30th potency depending on severity. Repeat as bleeding recurs.
		Uterine haemorrhage.	ONE 200th potency. Repeat as bleeding recurs.
	CARBO VEGETALIS	Slow oozing (e.g. from an abscess).	Repeat 6th potency hourly if needed.
	LACHESIS	Slow oozing (e.g. from abscess or ulcer).	Repeat 6th potency every hour.
		Black clotted (e.g. menses with much pain before flow starts).	ONE 30th potency

PRACTICE POINT

Once the bleeding has stopped it is important to continue to rest to allow the clot to form properly. Depending on the site, it may be useful to elevate the part. In some cases pressure on the wound may speed up clot formation but this is not usually necessary with Homoeopathy.

PROBLEM	REMEDY	SYMPTOMS	DOSE
BITES AND STINGS	*HYPERICUM*	Red, swelling, burning pain may shoot up limb, e.g. bee sting.	ONE 30th potency Repeat in higher potency if needed. Bathe the bee sting in baking soda.
	LEDUM	Swollen, numb, throbs. < heat.	ONE 30th potency Soak in vinegar if a wasp.
	HEPAR SULPHURIS	Red swollen, oozing as in dirty bite from horse fly (cleg).	ONE 30th potency. Repeat after 24 hours if needed.
	APIS MELLIFICA	Red, swollen, oedematous and shiny. Stinging pain > cold.	ONE 6-30th potency depending on severity.
	URTICA URENS	Where vesicles are formed and become itchy.	ONE 6-30th potency depending on severity.
	RHUS TOXICODENDRON	Itchy bites as in midgies.	Use cream as needed.

PRACTICE POINT

Use the lower potencies for children.

If you have to repeat a dose, repeat in the higher potency to get the effects of the venom out.

PROBLEM	REMEDY	SYMPTOMS	DOSE
BURNS	*CANTHARIS*	Scalds and where vesicles arise.	ONE 6-30th potency depending on severity. Repeat with return of pain.
		Severe burns with fluid loss.	ONE 30th potency Repeat plussed as needed. **Seek expert help.**
	HYPERICUM	Red, swollen, throbs and burns.	ONE 6-30th potency depending on severity.
		Should prevent sepsis where indicated. **Seek expert help.**	Start 30th potency and plus every 3-6 hours depending on severity.
	URTICA URENS	Scalds where vesicles are formed.	ONE 6-30th potency depending on severity. If need to, repeat plus.
		Sunburn – dry, flaky, stinging.	For sunburn use cream or boil young nettles in water for 20 minutes, add some honey and apply liquid (when cooled) to parts.
	BELLADONNA	Sunstroke – heat goes to head, dry – no sweat. Head feels full or enlarged. Can become delirious.	ONE 30~200~1M depending on severity.

> **PRACTICE POINT**
>
> Keep burns sterile – use Hypericum or Calendula or both as Hypercal on a dry dressing.
>
> Do not change the dressing in contact with the wound if there is skin loss, or danger of it. Use a second dressing and change this regularly. Apply Hypericum tincture 1:40 to the first dressing when disturbed.

PROBLEM	REMEDY	SYMPTOMS	DOSE
TOOTHACHE	*HYPERICUM*	Hot, swollen, throbbing. Shooting pains when touched or exposed to cold air.	ONE 30th potency Repeat with pain and **see dentist**.
	BELLADONNA	Hot swollen, throbbing pain shoot at touch. > cold.	ONE 30th potency Repeat with pain and **see dentist**.
	HEPAR SULPHURIS	Abscess – very sensitive to touch or draught. Throbs. Yellow discharge if visible.	Repeat 6-30th potency depending on severity every 3-6 hours.

READINGS

Harris Coulter	Homoeopathic Science and Modern Medicine	North Atlantic Books
Dorothy Sheppard	Homoeopathy for the First Aider	Health Science Press
George Vithoulkas	Homoeopathy and the New Man	Thorsons

THOUGHTS TO PONDER

The highest ideal of cure is rapid, gentle, and permanent restoration of the health, or removal and annihilation of the disease in its whole extent, in the shortest, most reliable, and most harmless way, on easily comprehensible principles.

> Para 2, The Organon of the Rational Art of Healing
> Samuel Hahnemann

He is likewise a preserver of health if he knows the things that derange health and cause disease, and how to remove them from persons in health.

> Para 4, The Organon of the Rational Art of Healing
> Samuel Hahnemann

Lesson 1

EXERCISE ON SYMPTOM PICTURES (page 18)

After breaking a leg

Ask what kind of pain (Sensation). Bruised pain is *Arnica*; shootings pains may need *Hypericum* but if pain on the periosteum of the bone (Location) it may be *Ruta* or *Symphytum*. If it is a scraping pain, it may be *Rhus toxicodendron*.

With any of the above there may be swelling. Redness tends to be *Arnica* whilst blueness may be *Ledum*. The *Arnica* patient may be bleeding. Internally this is bruising but ask also, or look to see, whether the bleeding is oozing or spurting.

Strange, Rare and Peculiar symptoms may be prickling along the bone in *Arnica* or around the wound in *Ledum*, or there may be a sensation of a lump as in *Symphytum*.

Then of course, a case is a patient. How are they experiencing the problem? Are they weeping, angry or irritated, or avoiding company?

With boils

Location may be a hair follicle with red swelling and pus as in *Rhus toxicodendron*. The sensation of this patient is great itchiness. They are also very irritable and angry.

When sensation predominates, burning and stinging may lead to *Tarantula* especially if the patient is very restless in a jerky way so they are difficult to pin down. As the situation deepens, there may be blueness around the boil.

Arnica is also blue but this patient is very sensitive to touch, even of their shirt collar – Modality. The location of the boil is often around the nose.

Hepar sulphuris boil is more often found on the neck. It is angry with a pustular head, the pus smells of old cheese, i.e. it is sour. In *Hepar sulphuris* the modality is emphasised as they are very, very sensitive to the slightest touch, even of the air in a draught. The pain may be described as stabbing (remember its stick-like sensation) and again the patient is extremely irritable.

Head injury

The *Arnica* patient will come up rapidly in a lump on the site of injury. This may look bruised. Bruised also describes the sensation. The pain may continue as a distant ache. In more serious situations they will float in and out of consciousness, answering you lucidly.

Gelsemium has a stupor with heavy eyes and pain at the back of the head that is better after they urinate and is << as the head is lowered when they lie down to sleep. They will tremble too. You will see this on any movement so they may want to be held closely.

Hypericum is distinguished by numbness. The head feels as if it buzzes. What this shows is nerve involvement.

Tooth extraction

Arnica is indicated by the swelling, the bruised look and the bruised aching pain. They may bleed profusely – it is best to take the *Arnica* before the extraction.

LESSON 2   First Aid with Homoeopathy II

First Aid Remedies II – *Sprains and Strains*

Aims: To understand the homoeopathic treatment of Sprains and Strains.
To learn more about the remedies *Rhus toxicodendron* and *Ruta graveolus*.
To find out more about the Law of Similars and how remedies are selected.
To find out more about the Vital Force and disease.
To understand the principles behind choosing the dose homoeopathically.

New key words in use:

Outer tube	the Minimum Dose	Time
Inner tube	succussion	Location
Middle tube	plussing	Sensation
resonance	the Collective Single Dose	Modality
the Single Dose	indicating symptom	Materia Medica
the Single Remedy	core symptoms	Repertory

Healing Connective Tissue

In the first lesson we saw how the organism acts holistically, as a unit, in circumstances of shock. To the Homoeopath this is a **General** response. The Vital Force has initiated an all-out offensive to preserve life. The pattern initiated is so common it becomes a process rather than a group of symptoms. It is a primary response. You have already learned that there is a hierarchy of importance in symptoms indicating greater or lesser disturbance. This hierarchy extends to tissues and organs. Vital organs such as heart, lungs, kidneys, liver, brain are essential to life. Minor organs such as eyes and ears show signs of disturbance before the Vital Force will allow interference with vital organs.

There are three types of tissue of differing importance to the Vital Force. These arise in order of formation in the embryo. In the first lesson, with wounds and burns, we were concerned mainly with epithelial tissue. This forms the outside of the body as skin and lines the respiratory and digestive tracts. As the skin it forms the outer tube – at some point in evolution, after the round egg shape, came the long worm-like shape with an outer tube and an inner tube, an epidermis and an endodermis. More evolved worms developed a middle muscular layer, a mesoderm. The form of these structures is present at some stage in the embryo and retained by the Vital Force as an order of importance. The structure is found unadulterated in the artery wall that has an outer layer, an inner lining layer and a middle muscular layer.

Why is this important? The healing of these layers is different. Disease of the middle layer, of mesoderm tissue, is much more serious. Mesoderm tissue includes bone, muscles, ligaments, cartilage, tendons, blood and heart. Have you noticed how difficult it is to cure fibrositis? How long does it takes to heal cartilage, or sprains and strains that affect tendons and ligaments, sometimes muscles? Have you noticed that rheumatism is usually a disease of old age that takes many years to arise?

The First Aid approach will therefore be slightly different. The remedy may need to be repeated in a lower dose, as healing is slower. Additional treatment may be needed to support the healing such as support in the form of a bandage or heat to encourage circulation so there is no build-up of congestants such as lactic acid that gives rise to stiffness. Massage may aid circulation too. Rest may be important. Healing will take place but now we see that there may be optimum conditions for it and we can act to promote these.

SPRAINS AND STRAINS

Usually when we suffer a sprain we have fallen and twisted an ankle pulling the tendon or we may have landed on the wrist wrenching ligaments connecting bones. Strains to muscles may occur when we have lifted something too heavy or at an awkward angle pulling on the muscle and its attachments. Maybe we have been overdoing it in the garden, or walked a little too far when not very fit, or have been carrying heavy suitcases on holiday, or cleaning out the attic, moving furniture around. With the sprain there is local swelling and inflammation with attendant pain. With a strain there is pain and stiffness and sometimes heat. Anyone can suffer a sprain or a strain. Some may produce similar symptoms to strain in the muscular aches of flu or as a form of rheumatism after exposure to cold and damp.

The remedy may be different depending on the Location whether muscles or tendons and ligaments are affected. Joints vary so the wrist has only ligaments and bones whilst the knee has a synovial capsule to protect it – it is encased in fluid. Around the ankle and the wrist the boniness means a different kind of pain Sensation as the periosteum (sensitive lining of the bone) is damaged. Let us look at the remedies that occur commonly in such cases.

Rhus toxicodendron is a main remedy of muscle and connective tissue. It is used in both sprains and strains. Its keynote Modality < *first movement,* > *continued movement* is found in almost all muscular strain. Can you remember when you struggled to keep the part moving after injury because you knew it was going to stiffen? Strained muscles are better kept moving so lactic acid does not build up. The *Rhus toxicodendron* patient is better for anything that improves circulation – rubbing, massage, heat. Indeed they are physically restless and will not be able to sleep for the need to keep moving. A special Modality < *lifting* gives a particular Location of this remedy as the deltoid muscle of the upper arm. So important is this location that another keynote is *miscarriage on lifting the arms*. < *grasping* or turning the wrist as in opening a door shows involvement of the muscles of the forearm. Another keynote of the remedy *as if the bone was scraped* is the Sensation that arises if the periosteum of the bone is affected and shows that this remedy can heal in such cases.

Because of its *affinity* with connective tissue this remedy will heal a tendon or reattach a ligament in a fraction of the time usually taken.

Because it is also an inflammatory remedy producing swelling, added to its interest in connective tissue, it becomes a very useful remedy in healing synovial joints such as the knee when these have been wrenched badly so they start to swell, become red and very hot.

Ruta graveoleus This remedy is almost indistinguishable from *Rhus toxicodendron*. It has the same *aetiology* of *cold, damp weather and over-exertion*. It is < *first movement and* > *continued movement, better for heat and massage*. The difference is the Location. *Ruta graveoleus* has a special affinity with small joints such as wrists where there is less muscle and tendon so it is more useful in sprains. Another affinity Location is the periosteum of the bone – it has bruised bone Sensation.

Arnica We have already mentioned how similar this remedy is to *Rhus toxicodendron*. It is < *first movement,* > *continued movement,* > *rubbing,* > *heat*. It also tends to keep moving to prevent stiffness and swelling. It is the better choice remedy where there is damage to surrounding soft tissue and the possibility of bruising. Because it has to do with integrity, you will find its Location is the back muscles supporting the uprightness of the spine. It has an affinity for back muscles. Where the bone is involved the Sensation is different – remember there is *prickling inwards*. Mentally both can be *irritable* but *Arnica* is less demanding; in fact they will send you away saying nothing is wrong.

Silicea has a profound effect on bone and connective tissue when these are *slow to heal* or there is a *weakness*. Its particular Location is the back and the ankle its affinity. These patients are always going over their ankle causing sprains. You may recognise them as *chilly, pale, weak debilitated types* who are prone to *glandular infections* and colds whereas *Rhus toxicodendron* and *Arnica* are ruddy and fiery.

Note: This last is more a constitutional remedy rather than a remedy of one-off accidents. This means the back weakness, for example, may result in curvature of the spine.

> **EXERCISE**
>
> Look at some joints in an anatomy and physiology textbook. Note how they are made up of bones, tendons and ligaments.
>
> Feel your wrist and ankle. Can you separate the bones and tendons?
>
> Find a First Aid book and practise bandaging wrists, ankle and knee. You can do those on yourself. Haven't you signed up for that First Aid course yet?

SELF TEST

1. Which remedy has most bruising?
2. Why is *Ruta graveoleus* best choice for hand injuries?
3. Which of the four remedies is not worse for first movement and better continued movement?
4. Which remedy has a scraping sensation on the bone?
5. Which remedy will tell you to go away?
6. Why do we bandage sprained ankles and wrists?
7. Why does the *Silicea* patient keep on spraining their ankles?
8. What does rubbing or massage achieve in strained muscles?
9. Why does *Rhus toxicodendron* help synovial joints?
10. *Rhus toxicodendron* has a special effect on the deltoid muscle and it also has the aggravation < lifting. What is the connection? You will need an anatomy and physiology textbook!

Check your answers by reviewing the text.

Rhus toxicodendron

This remedy comes from North America. Its common name is Poison Ivy. Here is a remedy you will see a great deal in First Aid situations or in rheumatic complaints. It has a profound effect on connective tissue but also works on the skin to produce hives. It is a remedy of *inflammation*.

Some people are so allergic to Poison Ivy that they will produce the typical hives and spots from one mile downwind! The 'hives' are red, angry and *itching*. Even in an inflammatory sore throat the *Rhus toxicodendron* patient is characterised by itch. Reactions to garden plants and other irritants may require *Rhus toxicodendron*. Some insect bites, eating strawberries or too many tomatoes (*foods rich in acids*) may produce the itching hives. The itch is caused by a histamine reaction under the skin. Thus this remedy can be used in many situations for which Antihistamine is the usual prescription. Where the reaction is more suppurative, the spot produced is *raised and red with a white pustular head*. This is typically found in chicken-pox for which *Rhus toxicodendron* is a common remedy.

This gives a clue to the action of *Rhus toxicodendron* in rheumatism. The metabolism is very acid. When muscles stiffen whether after overuse or in chronic rheumatism, there is a build-up of lactic acid as circulation does not take it away. Again this explains why *Rhus toxicodendron* is a specific for rheumatism which often has the symptoms:

> < cold, damp weather
>
> < first movement, > continued motion
>
> < rest, stiffens
>
> > rubbing or massage
>
> > heat.

The patient is so *physically restless* because they stiffen up if not moving. They *move about all night* and/or are so irritable and crotchety in the morning. They *wake up exhausted*. Rheumatism may be the result of a lifetime's abuse of alcohol or sugar so their metabolism is more acidic. With their red face and irritability, I see them as one of the crotchety old colonel remedies. I have an image of them waving their walking stick at a young rascal. Whilst they may be really jovial, they *fear being poisoned* so become anxious and apprehensive.

The stiffness may occur temporarily because they have been *lying on damp grass*, or because of overuse of muscles – going out for a long hill walk when they are out of condition. The knees are a favourite site of complaint after a hill walk that uses the knees, or after kneeling in the damp to cut the grass. The *synovial capsule swells* with excess protective fluid. On the outside this shows *red and hot*. There is an affinity for synovial joints and also for the *deltoid muscle*. The latter is often affected when they *lift something down from a shelf or hang out the washing*. This stretching up affects the womb so they may have a *miscarriage after reaching high*. Note that the womb is also muscle.

Now whilst the above is explicable in terms of chemistry under the skin or in the muscles, why should the symptoms appear predominantly on the *right side*? It is in such symptoms that we enter the **Individuality** of a homoeopathic remedy.

Numbness may occur or even *pins and needles*. It may be the remedy needed when overstretching produces pins and needles down the arms, or when overuse of a strimmer in the garden leads to pins and needles (*Hypericum* may be the better remedy due to jar of the nerves – see other symptoms). If we remember the earlier comments on chicken-pox, it may lead to another link. Chicken-pox in an adult more often leads to shingles which is an affliction of nerves. When the severe nerve pain is an excruciating itch and/or numbness and tingling, *Rhus toxicodendron* may be the best choice of remedy.

We usually see this remedy as a remedy of older people with their rheumatism but forget that it is a remedy of serious inflammatory conditions such as scarlet fever and rheumatic fever, both thankfully less common these days. However, they should remind us that this is a remedy of great violence in its action. It is easy to suppress symptoms with Homoeopathy if you repeat the dose and it is wise to remember here that rheumatism is a disease of heart and circulation. The Vital Force puts the disturbance out into the extremities to defend the heart. The end result of most rheumatism is heart disease. (See the section on assessing the action of the remedy below.) When the remedy is matched to the action of the Vital Force, it cures from the inside out, strengthening vital organs, possibly aggravating less vital organs or peripheries on the way.

The athletes who over-develop muscles end up with an enlarged heart. A keynote of the remedy is *dreams of great exertion (and wakes exhausted)* because they have been moving about all night. There is so much physical movement in the remedy. Where this is stifled, activity still continues so the irritability may go to the head to produce High Blood Pressure. Bringing the patient back to physical exercise frequently helps without medication. The tension eventually reaches its opposite, the second action of the medicine, producing a slackness that is visible as oedema – Angiotensin 1 is converted in the muscles to Angiotensin 2 that acts with Aldosterone in the kidneys to regulate fluid in the body. In First Aid we saw this in swollen synovial capsules.

In acute ailments it appears as swollen glands or swollen skin problems. In older weaker constitutions it is seen in swollen extremities which are better for exercise in the early days. If it continues through to chronic rheumatic disease it may end up with congestive heart disease where the swollen extremities affect the functioning of the heart and lead to a different kind of High Blood Pressure that is more difficult to cure because the parts are weakened. The dreams at this point are of *drowning*. Is it not interesting how the unconsciousness reflects the state of the body? The mental state may now be *despondency* that leads them to suicidal thoughts ... by drowning!

Modalities – AS above but also < cold air so their cough may start up, even putting a hand out from the covers. A common aetiology is *after getting soaked*. < *before stormy weather* reminds of the rheumatic who knows it will rain soon!

> **EXERCISE**
>
> I have marked out the keynotes in italics above and will continue to do so in all other remedies so you can learn the signature tune of the remedies.
>
> Can you find which symptoms of Individuality belong under the following headings?
>
> LOCATION
>
> SENSATION
>
> MODALITY
>
> Aetiology is TIME. What examples can you find above?
>
> Can you separate the symptoms into Strange, Rare and Peculiar, Mental and Emotional, General and Particular?
>
> Some answers at the end of this lesson will help you.

Ruta gravoleus

This is the herb Rue. It shows so much similarity to *Rhus toxicodendron* that they are hard to tell apart.

It has the same aggravations from *cold, damp* and *over-exertion*. It is ameliorated by *motion* and by *rubbing*, so it is restless also. It has the same *quarrelsome* nature but they *fear they are being deceived* where *Rhus toxicodendron* fears being poisoned. This gives a different feel when you are with them. *Rhus toxicodendron's* fear pushes you out and away from them, similar to *Arnica* but the *Ruta graveoleus* patient imposes upon you. The energy is different and part of the skill of the Homoeopath to identify. It is this energy that becomes the **Essence**. We will talk more of this later.

The art of the Homoeopath is also in recognising that although the symptoms may be the same there is a different emphasis, e.g. in Location, Sensation or Modality. This may be so subtle it takes years of training to see it. Both *Rhus toxicodendron* and *Ruta graveoleus* have an affinity with connective tissue but *Ruta graveoleus* has a particular affinity with tendons and muscles, etc, hence it is more specific to the treatment of hands and small joints that have fewer ligaments. Such joints also tend to be bony and bones are covered in periosteum that is a fibrous connective tissue rich in nerves. *Ruta graveoleus* is more emphasised in the severe pain when the periosteum is damaged. As *Calendula* helps restore the integrity of epithelial tissue so *Ruta graveoleus* cures ganglions and nodes on connective tissue, e.g. around the wrist.

There is a distinct *blunt plug sensation*. The ear pain is described as of a *blunt piece of wood* – note how this is different from *Arnica's* sensation *as if hit by a blunt piece of wood*. Another similarity to *Arnica* is the *bruised, lame feeling, especially in parts lain on*.

There is so little to differentiate this remedy from *Rhus toxicodendron*. The bladder is tensed so feels full even after urinating. This is a deeper symptom in an organ so you may not see it in a First Aid situation. Remember, do not discount a remedy because a symptom is missing unless that symptom really is central to the remedy at that phase in its development of a symptom picture – what I will later call a **core symptom**. *Ruta graveoleus* is a useful remedy in rectal prolapse after passing a stool, or when the legs give way when first rising up from sitting or lying, but you may see neither of these in a First Aid situation because this is the chronic rheumatic symptom picture.

There is little of the inflammation of *Rhus toxicodendron* except in the eyes that *burn like balls of fire* from overuse or stain. *Rhus toxicodendron* similarly affects the eyes but usually in an acute syndrome where the first symptom is in the muscles or in iritis that accompanies arthritis.

EXERCISE

Make up four columns labelled:

STRANGE, RARE AND PECULIAR	MENTAL AND EMOTIONAL	GENERAL	PARTICULAR

Allocate the symptoms above to the appropriate column.

You will find some help with this at the end of the lesson.

SELF TEST

Mark the following TRUE or FALSE:

1. *Rhus toxicodendron* is a good remedy for eye strain. ....
2. *Ruta graveoleus* has a lame bruised feeling after getting wet on a cold day. ....
3. In *Ruta graveoleus* the fullness of the bladder is relieved after urinating. ....
4. *Rhus toxicodendron* is useful for shingles where there is an itch. ....
5. Both remedies feel poisoned. ....
6. The *Rhus toxicodendron* spot is white with a red top. ....
7. Stiffness is caused by a build-up of lactic acid in muscle tissue. ....
8. Both remedies are physically restless in the night. ....
9. *Ruta graveoleus* dreams of great exertion in the night. ....
10. If miscarriage threatens after hanging out the washing, *Rhus toxicodendron* may help. ....

Check the answers by reviewing the text.

THE LAW OF SIMILARS

This is the most fundamental law in Homoeopathy from which it gets its name – like cures like. You have heard of *the hair of the dog that bit you* saying that translates as what caused the ailment can relieve it. The effects of too much alcohol the night before may be relieved by another dose. Smokers know that the thick claustrophobic feeling in the chest is relieved first thing in the morning by their first cigarette of the day. Withdrawal symptoms from lack of coffee may disappear after a few cups. This well-known effect is not quite the same as Homoeopathy because we do not take exactly the same substance. We take something *similar* that can produce a similar symptom picture.

The power of Homoeopathy rests on its ability to affect the Vital Force. In Homoeopathy we accept that every medicine is a medicine because of its ability to affect health but that need not be for the good. Many homoeopathic remedies are violent poisons, e.g. the snake venoms, Atropine Belladonna, Nux vomica that contains strychnine, Arsenicum is arsenic oxide. The Homoeopath accepts that every medicine has two actions, the first being opposite to the second. There are no side effects in Homoeopathy because we take both the actions of the remedy into consideration. Indeed when we give a homoeopathic remedy, we understand that it introduces an artificial disease. Some will say Homoeopathy is similar to vaccination because of this. If the remedy introduced can create a similar symptom picture to that from which the organism already suffers, then the remedy will impose its own picture *if it is strong enough*. We know this has happened when the *aggravation* occurs after the remedy. The symptoms from which the patient is suffering get worse [1].

In a First Aid situation where the Vital Force is healthy, the aggravation may only last a few minutes. In a constitutional case it may take days to appear and go on for several more days. Some Homoeopaths do not feel cure is possible without the aggravation. Others like myself feel that there is an optimum point or balance where the remedy is strong enough to take over without too much further disturbance. The key to the strength of the remedy is the potency. The Homoeopath will select a potency to match the energy needed for the remedy to take over the symptom picture of the patient.

---

[1] There is a fallacy afoot that horrifies me that I hear from so many other alternative practitioners. It is that the symptoms get worse after the remedy and that it is good. The symptoms that get worse after the remedy are dispersing the disease from within out according to Hering's Laws of Cure, following the path of least resistance and operating through channels and drains that are either natural or are temporarily active in acute cases. Through potency usually the Homoeopath can control this aggravation within bearable limits to the patient. Aggravations are not haphazard but predictable. Homoeopathy is very precise. More of this later.

I like to use the harmony of music to explain it further. Notes in a harmonic series if sounded will awaken the other notes in the series even when not struck, e.g. the over tones. Another model to explain the process is the coil in a car or television. A car does not run on 12 volts. A television does not run on 240 volts. The coil is two coils one inside the other at a critical distance so the spark jumps the gap and is massively increased in voltage. The distance apart is as critical as the degree of similarity of a homoeopathic remedy. Too close and there will be aggravation with no amelioration. Too far apart and you lose the resonance.

If you understand this principle you have the fundamental basis of Homoeopathy. Homoeopathy introduces the spark that energises the system. If you need to keep sparking, you need to check the system.

Now we need to find the symptom picture of remedies.

More about Provings

The efficiency of Homoeopathy depends largely on how accurately we match the symptom picture of the remedy to that of the patient. The symptoms of illness are produced by the Vital Force in the process of cure so the remedy must be able to produce these symptoms to enhance the outward flow of the symptoms to bring about cure.

To find the nature of a remedy we take it in a **proving**. Healthy people with no disturbance are given the remedy. We do not use animals because they cannot speak and tell us the subtle subjective sensations. We do not use sick people because they are already producing a pattern that would conflict with what we want to see of the remedy.

There is a group of provers of different ages and sex. Before they take the remedy they note down for two weeks any symptoms they may have. This forms an individual base line. The provers are kept away from any stress and asked to desist from any intoxicants, etc that might interfere with the symptoms to be produced by the remedy. They do not talk to anyone except their supervisor. When symptoms appear they have to try different postures, etc to find the modalities.

Once the prover starts to produce symptoms the remedy is stopped. One of the most important instructions in the proving is not to restart taking the remedy after it has been stopped because until the symptoms appear fully we do not know what effect the remedy has had on the Vital Force. When the Vital Force has been disturbed by a remedy it will go on producing symptoms, sometimes for months afterwards, until it has restored harmony. When repeating the dose it is as if the Vital Force has been held down under the water. When the dosage is stopped it bounces up and starts the process of rebalancing. This is important to know when you repeat the dose – **there may be no reaction until you stop taking the medicine**. That is why most Homoeopaths give only a single dose of the remedy then wait to see what the Vital Force is going to do next. The Homoeopath listens and follows the guidance of the Vital Force which speaks through the symptoms to tell us what is happening to it.

There are over 2000 remedies that have been proved over a period of almost 200 years. Some have been proved very thoroughly, others not so. The style of the actual proving has changed over time to achieve more accuracy and precision. Sometimes only a single pill in high potency was given. At other times a lower potency was repeated until some change was affected then no more pills were taken.

When we take the remedy there is an order to the appearance of the pattern of symptoms that will be repeated in the sick patient. Each remedy has its own unique pattern putting emphasis according to its own Individuality. This Individuality is also reflected in the patient. The full proving of a remedy will contain symptoms from all the groups – Strange, Rare and Peculiar, Mental and Emotional, General and Particular. We will see Location, Sensation and Modality as the pattern of symptoms develops in the prover. When we add all these elements together, the symptom picture of each remedy is unique.

Samuel Hahnemann, the founder of modern Homoeopathy, started doing provings almost 200 years ago, yet today we still use his remedies. Indeed homoeopathic remedies are not discarded and do not change over time. Once we know their symptom pattern we can use them whenever that pattern arises in a sick person. The symptom pictures of remedies are gathered in huge tomes called *materia medicas*. They may be ordered in dictionaries called **repertories**. The Repertory most in use today was created at the turn of this century by J. T. Kent.

Specifics

You have heard me use this term in the case of *Arnica* in head injury, *Calendula* and epithelial tissue, *Rhus toxicodendron* and connective tissue, and *Hypericum* and tetanus. Despite having already met four of them, specifics are rare in Homoeopathy so need special attention.

We do not prescribe for disease but for each unique symptom picture. However, sometimes the symptom picture of a remedy is so close to a particular disease pattern or defensive process that it very frequently cures that disease pattern or speeds rebalance through that defence mechanism. This remedy is called a **specific**. The Individuality of the remedy matches the disease peculiarities as expressed in the symptoms. So specifics are the closest Homoeopaths come to routine prescriptions.

> **EXERCISE**
>
> I will not ask you to take a homoeopathic remedy in a proving because we seldom see our own symptom changes at subtle levels so need outside supervision. If you are using this textbook in a study group with an experienced Homoeopath that might be a possibility! However, it may be a useful exercise for you to keep a prover's diary for two weeks. Write down all the symptoms that occur to you. Do a regular check every 2-3 hours. You will be amazed at the different view of your health that arises.

More about Dosage

There is always more to learn about this even when you have been in practise for a number of years so here is a little more to think about.

The Single Remedy

This fundamental law of Homoeopathy is very simple. When we do provings we explore only one remedy at a time so we do not know what happens when you mix remedies. Remember this is physics, not chemistry; if you mix colour pigment you get a different colour from when you mix light.

The Minimum Dose

Samuel Hahnemann discovered that the medicine can interfere with the rate of cure. By reducing the dose he came to an optimum balance. Later he went much further. He discovered the process of **potentisation**. Not only did he dilute the dose, he also succussed it. One of his friends was Lavoisier, the great scientist who discovered oxygen. Goodness knows how he stumbled on the process of succussion and dilution so long before quantum physics. We now know that water retains the memory of the substance. We also now know that DNA is composed of water tubules that retain the memory and it appears that it is these that the homoeopathic remedy resonates with, hence a homoeopathic remedy acts holistically to affect the whole organism.

Paul Callinan from Australia demonstrated that water containing the remedy frozen at −200° Centigrade would consistently repeat the same snowflake pattern identifiable with the remedy. What I found most interesting about his work was as the remedy was further diluted, i.e. as the potency was increased, the pattern became clearer and clearer. To the Homoeopath these higher dilutions contain more energy and have a wider effect on the symptom picture – we could say a deeper effect on the Vital Force.

The Practical Application – Potency

The Vital Force is invisible. We see only the effects of its actions in symptoms so the role of a homoeopathic remedy is to start or speed up the process of cure. The Vital Force knows exactly what is out of harmony and sets out to restore order in the quickest and most safe way. It knows where the blocks are; it knows where the drains and channels of flow are – we do not, therefore it is a fundamental part of Homoeopathy in helping the Vital Force to sound the tuning fork only once then watch the change in the symptom picture to find out what is happening.

We also try to judge the amount of energy needed to resonate with the disturbance hence sometimes I have chosen a 30th potency. Where there is greater disturbance, I have recommended a higher potency, 200th or 1M. Where there is less energy or we know there is more physical dross to move, I have suggested a 6th potency and then to repeat it. The potency is the speed at which the Vital Force can move or needs to move. In the case of burns where the healthy body is curing, I have suggested a 30th potency, but when pain returns to indicate another dose, I have suggested **plussing** the remedy – this is to put it back into dilution then to succuss it before each repeat dose to slightly up (increase) the potency. Where the patient's health is at a delicate stage as in a burns case, we do not want the repeat sounding of the tuning fork. The resonance needs to be slightly higher in octave to raise the vibrations of the Vital Force higher.

That is an interesting topic. Energy indicated by rate of vibration changes through octaves, as we see in music, the more refined energy being in higher octaves so light is much more refined than sound! How refined is a human organism? Certainly when health is low we speak of being down, we are slowed down and duller in consciousness.

When the patient is less fragile and the symptoms return, we up the potency if there is no physical alterations needed, or as in the head injury we really want to move obstruction fast. There is no real danger in upping the potency that has worked but keep in mind that Homoeopathy is not about removing symptoms, it is about curing. How is cure represented in the symptom pattern? We will speak of Hering's Laws of Cure shortly. If we give too much energy the patient will simply do a proving of the remedy and such extra symptoms will wear off quickly in a few hours or a day or two. However, where the patient is more fragile, as in the burns case, we raise the potency slowly through the plussing process. We do not want to divert healing energy into a proving!

The potencies available reflect a harmonic shift of octave – 6, 30, 200, 1M (1000), 10M, LM, CM, MM.

The Practical Application – Symptoms

Always I like to define **indicating symptoms** that reflect which symptoms must go. I also call these the **core symptoms** of a constitutional case. These are often pains in First Aid situations. It could be swelling, redness or fluid loss. The keynote symptoms are usually the core of the remedy's action so should go after the remedy or return if more of the remedy is needed. Needless to say, when another remedy is needed the keynote symptoms change! When repeating a remedy in a 6th potency it is important to have a clear idea of what is to be cured and some indicating symptom to measure, or to monitor that cure because you cannot go on repeating a homoeopathic remedy without getting to its second action. If you miss the point of cure, the second action is that the patient gets worse again. I was horrified when one patient spoke of taking *Arnica 6* 2-3 times per day after his operation. He raved as to how quickly his operation cut had healed. Two weeks later he could not understand why he had boils all along his nicely healing scar. *Arnica* is also a remedy of boils! He had gone beyond the Vital Force's healing process to deflect its attention to other matters.

In the tables I have tried to give you a clearer idea of the relationship between the symptom and the potency, of how the severity is indicated by the depth of the symptom picture – where depth is the depth of disturbance of the Vital Force.

SUMMARY

PROBLEM	REMEDY	SYMPTOMS	DOSE
SPRAINS AND STRAINS	RHUS TOXICODENDRON	Hot, swollen, aching, bruised. < first movement, > continued movement, > rubbing, > heat ARM < lifting, < grasping Restless, dreams of exertion as if the bone scrapped.	ONE 30th potency after the event and repeat as pain recurs. In older injuries or where there is less vitality repeat the 6th potency every 3-6 hours and use the swelling as an indicating symptom.
	RUTA GRAVEOLEUS	Location – wrists and ankles. < first movement, > continued movement, > rubbing, > heat Bruised sensation or severe gnawing pains as periosteum involved.	ONE 30th potency after the event and repeat as pain recurs. In older injuries or where there is less vitality repeat the 6th potency every 3-6 hours. Use pain or swelling as an indicating symptom.
	ARNICA	Bruised pain < first movement, > continued movement, > rubbing, > heat. Stiffness sets in quickly if do not move. Surrounding tissue may be bruised. Prickling pain inwards if bone affected. Broken bones.	ONE 30th potency Repeat as needed when pain recurs.
	SILICEA	Patient chilly. Location back and ankles. Tremble with weakness.	Repeat 6th potency every 6 hours. Use trembling as an indicating symptom.

RHUS TOXICODENDRON	STRANGE, RARE AND PECULIAR	MENTAL AND EMOTIONAL	GENERAL
TIME	Spontaneous abortion on reaching high.		Eating acid foods such as strawberries and tomatoes.
LOCATION			Extremities. Right side.
SENSATION	As if the bone were scraped.	Fear of being poisoned.	Itching Restless
MODALITY			< first movement, > continued movement, > rubbing. Heat

EXERCISE

Once of the most difficult things to do is to discard information. In the table above we have selected out some information. Construct a similar table for *Ruta graveoleus* and *Arnica*.

You are learning to isolate significant homoeopathic information.

READINGS

A little more reading around the homoeopathic remedies studied will help you see into the Homoeopath's magic garden.

E. B. Nash — Leaders in Homoeopathic Therapeutics — Jain Publishers, India
This will illustrate the use of keynotes in common acute ailments.

H. C. Allen — Keynotes and Characteristics with Comparisons — Jain Publishers, India
This illustrates the different grades of symptoms using different typefaces. Bold type symptoms are found in most provings so we expect to find them prominent in the patient's symptom picture if we want to use that remedy. Italic type symptoms are common in the provings of the remedy but not present in all provers. Ordinary type was present in just a few provers but we know it has some clinical worth from experience.

THOUGHTS TO PONDER

There is, in the interior of man, nothing morbid that is curable and no invisible alteration that is curable which does not make itself known to the accurately observing physicians by means of morbid signs and symptoms – an arrangement in perfect conformity with the infinite goodness of the all-wise Preserver of human life.

Para 14, The Organon of the Rational Art of Healing
Samuel Hahnemann

The human body appears to admit of being much more powerfully affected in its health by medicines (partly because we have the regulation of the dose in our own power) than by natural morbid stimuli – for natural diseases are cured and overcome by suitable medicines.

Para 30, The Organon of the Rational Art of Healing
Samuel Hahnemann

Lesson 2

SYMPTOMS EXERCISES (pages 39, 40)

Rhus toxicodendron

Time	< overuse, < lying on damp grass, < getting soaked
Location	synovial joints, hair follicles, deltoid muscle
Sensation	angry itching, numbness
Modality	< damp cold, < first movement > continued movement, > rubbing, > heat, < lifting
Strange, Rare and Peculiar	Dreams of exertion and wakes exhausted
Mental/Emotional	Fear they will be poisoned, dreams of drowning
General	Restless, right sided
Particular	Raised, red eruptions with a pustular head

Ruta graveolas

STRANGE, RARE AND PECULIAR	MENTAL AND EMOTIONAL	GENERAL	PARTICULAR
Blunt plug sensations	Fear they are being deceived	< cold damp	> rubbing
Bladder full even after urinating		< over-exerting	Rectal prolapse after passing stool
Eyes burn like balls of fire			Legs give way after rising from a seat

LESSON 3   Headaches

Aims: To understand the homoeopathic treatment of headaches.
To know the difference between tension, sinus, bilious headaches and migraines - neuralgic headaches.
To recap the value that the Homoeopath puts on symptoms.
To understand the difference between an exciting cause and a modality.
To understand the difference between an exciting and a maintaining cause.
To understand the homoeopathic view of an acute illness.
To study the relationship of an acute illness to the constitutional case.
To study the remedies *Nux vomica*, *Pulsatilla* and *Bryonia*.

New keywords used in text:
Maintaining cause
exciting cause
acute
chronic

concomitant symptoms
susceptibility
predisposition
repertorising

What are Headaches?

Pain in the head is usually a local symptom that the Homoeopath calls a **particular symptom**. It is seldom an incident in itself unless caused by something like a severe blow to the head. Usually it is related to other health issues so, although the Homoeopath may look for an immediate **acute** remedy, the overall general health needs attention. We call this working constitutionally, i.e. on the constitutional case which Hahnemann called the **chronic** case.

Sometimes the head pain symptoms cannot be separated from the constitutional symptom picture, for example when caused by a tumour or high blood pressure, or even rheumatism in the bones of the skull. We will not deal with such headaches here. Migraines proper are a debility of the nervous system. They come into our remit here when they are caused by nervous strain that is then a **maintaining cause**. When part of the constitutional picture, headache may appear before menstruation or at menopause (Time). As part of a larger constitutional symptom picture, the whole needs treated constitutionally to get deeper relief. Before menstruation or at menopause then become General **modalities**.

FOUR TYPES OF HEADACHE

Our world today is full of stress and over-stimulation of the nervous system – stand in a street and look around you to see the multi-coloured hoardings, the flashy shop windows and displays within shops, to hear the noise of traffic and people and feel the vibration of music in most shops. Leisure? What do you do? TV, film, disco? Film makers today talk about an impact every 2-3 minutes to keep the viewer's attention. For *attention* read alertness of the nervous system. Job? Time boundaries, schedules to finish, rush, hassle travelling to work, what and where is lunch, closed in, noisy buildings, people you would not normally choose to be around? Life today is very different for the nervous system than even 30-40 years ago. Is it surprising therefore that it is weakened leading to neuralgic pain in the head and visual disturbances, with sensitivity to light and noise? The **migraine headache** appears more common in these days. It is often above one eye and one sided. It may have numbness or be described as excruciating. Often there is clumsiness, dropping things or the person is prone to trip and knock things over. Memory or speech may be affected showing the involvement of the brain.

A **tension headache** is usually found in the muscles at the back of the head, the nape of the neck, where the patient has continuously contracted the muscles so they go into spasm. It often extends to the shoulders or over the top to sit above the eyes where it throbs sharply or, more often, feels tight. It could be described as like a band or a vice. Such headaches are better for rest.

A **bilious headache** is one of congestion where the action of the liver is insufficient to remove all the toxins that are the product of catabolism. The head may feel heavy, consciousness dull. There may be a feeling of pressure at the top of the head or all over. They may feel the head would burst. The sensation is often throbbing. Lying down and heat do not help as these increase the flow and therefore exposure to more toxins. This patient is often nauseous. They may even feel better after they have vomited. If the eyes are affected, it is with a sore pain. Vision may be occluded with black spots that indicate the poor action of the liver.

The **sinus headache** is usually frontal over the eyes, or cheekbones, where there are sinuses in the bones of the skull. Either there is catarrh there or dryness so they feel full and heavy or stuffy. Drainage is affected by gravity so the sensations are worse stooping or lying down. Sometimes the sensations are worse for sudden movement like turning the head quickly – when this happens the ears may be involved with catarrh. The pain is an ache or a dull throb. The patient describes a fullness. They are sensitive to dry heat, and usually better in the open air where the sinuses drain as coryza.

So many of us have headaches. There are so many remedies but there is much Individuality in the symptoms. We will look more closely at this shortly. First an exercise.

EXERCISE

Describe the type of headache **you** suffer from.

Can you gather a few more headache types from your family?

Check that you have *full symptoms* with Time, Location, Sensation and Modality.

You may find another group of symptoms in your list, Concomitant symptoms. **Concomitant symptoms** occur at the same time as other symptoms. An example here could be *nausea* or *dizziness*. *Visual disturbance* is commonly a concomitant symptom in migraine headaches.

ANATOMY AND PHYSIOLOGY

The head is one of the first areas that show something is not quite right with our health. Why? Let us look at the Anatomy and Physiology.

The head is particularly prone to pain because of its structure and function. It has a bony box protecting the centre of the nervous system. Within its influence are the sense organs receiving impressions of sound and light, smell and taste. The lower part of the head has openings to the respiratory and digestive systems, passage being assisted and regulated by a hinged jaw. The bones of the box are penetrated by hollows called sinus. Problems occasionally arise here when the epithelial lining tissue over-secretes mucus causing drainage problems. This gives rise to the sinus headache which is often aggravated and ameliorated by changing the position of the head, or by heat or cold that increases or decreases the flow of secretions.

The internal construction of the box is characterised by lack of space. The box is rigid preventing expansion in inflammation or injury. Swelling within the box is dangerous because it puts pressure on the vulnerable brain. Bleeding within the box has the same danger as the brain responds to pressure by altering its function so consciousness is altered or even absent. The brain is protected by two membranes, the meninges, that are further cushioned with fluid filling the space between them. Thus as we leap about, the brain does not rattle off the bony box but is protected by the same mechanism as the baby in the womb, i.e. fluid. Inflammation in this area, meningitis, may increase the fluid bringing pressure to bear on the precious brain. Meningitis may also involve increase in the cerebro-spinal fluid filling the space around the spinal cord and the ventricles within the brain. Injury to the head is serious because the damage may vary depending on the locality, bruising and bleeding and the pressure arising out of these. This is why *Arnica* is important in head injury – it stops bleeding and bruising.

The role of the brain and nervous system is consciousness and control. Well supplied with nerves whose function is sensation, pain is easily perceived in the head. The neuralgic headache, or migraine, well illustrates this when pain is tearing, excruciating as only nerve pain can be. Numbness associated with many migraines may arise from over-stimulation and burn-out of nerve receptors. Visual disturbance in migraines also shows the effect of nerve dysfunction. When dizziness and nausea are involved the autonomic nervous system has been stimulated. Connections here are through the hindbrain and cerebellum which controls co-ordination of voluntary muscles – dysfunction gives rise to clumsiness. Mixing up words and forgetfulness that occurs with some migraines shows some effect on the memory and language centres in the brain.

The most frequent changes in the head environment occur from the composition of the blood that varies easily as blood is a transport medium. In headaches we are particularly interested in the debris produced by metabolic breakdown, catabolism. Of course, the content of this debris varies from day to day and from individual to individual depending on lifestyle, diet, habit and constitutional make-up, e.g. the individual with a diabetic diathesis will differ from another with a rheumatic diathesis. Each of us may vary daily depending on how much alcohol we have consumed or how much tobacco smoke we have been exposed to. The key is the efficiency of the liver in taking the toxins out of the blood. It may depend on just how much work we give the liver to do hence heavy foods like cheese that are difficult to digest often produce headaches. Because the liver excretes oestrogen from the body, its role is increased prior to the menses so women often suffer headaches before their monthly period. The headache arising here is the bilious headache. Dullness of consciousness arises from the sluggish flow. Worse stooping tells us it is a congestive headache. Worse heat is common as this increases the blood flow.

The tension headache occurs in the muscles at the back of the neck when we steel ourselves to get on with something, or when we bear up under pressure. We grasp our body tightly in order to perform, or overperform, or push ourselves. The continuous tension causes unnatural contraction of the muscles. That may extend down into the shoulders but frequently the tension rises to settle over the eyes where we contract the brows in a frown. The contraction explains why this headache is often experienced as a tightness or cramp.

> **EXERCISE**
>
> Look at the structure of the head in an Anatomy and Physiology textbook.

The Symptom Picture of a Headache

What we have looked at above is the *common* symptom picture based on an understanding of the Anatomy and Physiology. This does not enable us to select a homeopathic remedy although it does enable us to see what needs cured in terms of the five pillars of health, i.e. the maintaining causes. When we have isolated the maintaining causes that affect health in general we can then find the individual causes or symptoms that indicate the homoeopathic remedy.

Maintaining Causes

Maintaining causes are bad health habits. When removed they will enable vitality to be restored automatically. For example, when we have a tension headache we need to reduce the stress levels to stop further damage then relax to enable the muscles to let go the spasm. Until this has occurred cure is not possible. We need to leave the stressful environment, change our attitude to that boss or bit of work, slow down and unburden ourselves. You will find a couple of exercises below to relieve strain in this area at the back of the head.

In the case of the bilious headache we need to reassess the intake of food, drink and air. Is it too much or too little? What is the quality needed to function efficiently? Some foods are poisonous – alcohol, tea, coffee. Others over-stimulate the digestive system and may even affect the nerves – fats, spices, sugars. Some foods may only affect in quantities. Often these food affect anyone, each and every one of us, so are maintaining causes. Others affect different people in different ways. This last group moves us into individual **susceptibility** that becomes the **exciting cause**.

Exciting Causes

To find the homoeopathic remedy we need Individuality; irrespective of the cause we each produce a unique pattern of symptoms. Included in Individuality, but separate, is that to which each one of us is susceptible, the resonance that responds to cause and produces points of change in the symptom picture. The Homoeopath will speak of the underlying chronic pattern of weaknesses that we inherit.

Our family might have heart problems, or be prone to bowel problems, etc. From these weaknesses, or *predispositions*, arise the exciting causes. With heart problems our family is very sensitive to bad news. All people may ultimately be affected by bad news but our family is so sensitive it becomes an exciting cause. After all, few are struck dumb as our Jeannie was on hearing her son had a terrible accident. And John, he has never recovered from the shock of being made redundant. He still has nightmares, five years later. The family with bowel problems may speak of sensitivity to wheat or milk, or individuals within it may not be able to wait for food. One may develop headaches if they do not eat on time. Another may become very aggressive and violent if kept waiting in a restaurant for more than five minutes.

The exciting cause links the headache to the underlying constitution. Usually we are aware that *our* headache always follows the same pattern of symptoms and has a recognised trigger.

EXERCISES FOR TENSION RELEASE

1. It is not easy to let go of tensed muscles. Massage helps. However, we could draw our attention to it by further contracting then releasing the muscles.

2. Lift the shoulders very very slowly, pull the head down into the shoulders and tighten then release just as slowly. Do this three times at least.

3. If pain is in the shoulders, you could add another exercise after 2. Rotate the shoulders slowly one at a time forwards three times then backwards three times.

4. Rest.

5. Where do you feel tense now? Pay attention.

6. If still tense in the neck muscles, bend the head forward slowly then back, then to the left then to the right side. Slowly. Then rotate the neck three times one way then the other way.

7. Rest.

In the Repertory you will find over 100 pages with different headache symptoms. Below are a few symptoms of Individuality that may lead you more quickly to a remedy. Remember, we never go on one symptom alone but put it into the Total Symptom Picture.

Some Exciting Causes

Time – what happened at the start that put the Vital Force off key? Here is a list of exciting causes that you will easily come across and that feature many of the remedies we are studying. It will give you an idea of what the Homoeopath looks for in a symptom picture, that golden Strange, Rare and Peculiar symptom that leads us swiftly to the remedy.

Hot bathing	*Belladonna, Calcarea carbonica*
After a blow to the head	*Arnica, Hypericum*
Catarrh suppressed	*Belladonna, Lachesis*
Constipation	*Bryonia, Nux vomica*
Damp room, sleeping in excitement	*Bryonia, Belladonna, Lycopodium, Natrum muriaticum, Nux vomica, Phosphorus, Pulsatilla, Staphisagria*
After exposure to cold winds	*Aconite, Nux vomica, Rhus toxicodendron, Silicea*
Straining the eyes	*Calcarea carbonica, Lycopodium, Natrum muriaticum, Phosphorus, Ruta graveoleus, Silicea*
Worse fasting	*Lycopodium, Phosphorus, Silicea, Sulphur*
Worse after fright	*Aconite, Ignatia, Nux vomica, Rhus toxicodendron*
Since grief	*Ignatia, Natrum muriaticum, Pulsatilla, Staphisagria*
After a haircut	*Belladonna*
After ironing	*Bryonia, Sepia*
After lifting	*Calcarea carbonica*
Worse strong light	*Gelsemium*
Worse menstruation	*Bryonia, Calcarea carbonica, Lachesis, Natrum muriaticum, Pulsatilla, Sepia*
Worse menopause	*Bryonia, Calcarea carbonica, Lachesis, Sepia*
Nervous exhaustion	*Gelsemium, Ignatia, Nux vomica, Silicea*
Worse running	*Bryonia, Ignatia, Natrum muriaticum, Nux vomica, Pulsatilla*
Comes with sea sickness	*Cocculus*
After sexual intercourse	*Calcarea carbonica, Lycopodium, Phosphorus, Sepia, Silicea*
Sleep loss	*Cocculus, Nux vomica*
After getting soaked	*Belladonna* (head), *Dulcamara, Pulsatilla* (feet), *Rhu toxicodendron*
After exposure to the sun	*Belladonna, Natrum muriaticum, Pulsatilla*
After exposure to tobacco	*Gelsemium, Ignatia, Nux vomica*

Some Food Causes

Time or Modality – these are not necessarily *'allergies'*. In Homoeopathy, it is accepted that each person will have *susceptibility*. Each individual will have their own trigger points. This is not the same as the hyperactive state today called *allergic*. Similarly, because each of us has different metabolism and life style, we each have modalities to which we respond. The difference between Time and Modality is quite subtle. The first causes an acute symptom picture because it disturbs the Vital Force. Once in force it has to run through to the crisis that resolves the disturbance. A Modality affects the vitality so there is slower build up, like a maintaining cause, and any lessening of the modality will bring relief.

Worse after consuming alcohol	*Bryonia, Gelsemium, Lachesis, Nux vomica, Pulsatilla, Sepia*
beer	*Bryonia, Sepia*
cheese	*Arsenicum, Bryonia, Nux vomica, Rhus toxicodendron*
coffee	*Chamomilla, Ignatia, Nux vomica, Pulsatilla*
cold food	*Dulcamara, Pulsatilla*
fatty food	*Ipecacuanha. Pulsatilla, Sepia*
ice cream	*Pulsatilla*
rich food	*Bryonia, Ipecacuanha, Nux vomica, Pulsatilla, Sepia*
red wine	*Lycopodium*

Location

Different remedies have their favourite location. Patients are inclined to get pain in the same localities so they can recognise it as *their* headache.

Frontal extending to the eyes, root of nose	*Aconite, Bryonia, Hepar sulphuris, Ignatia, Lachesis*
Frontal extending to the occiput and spine	*Bryonia, Gelsemium, Nux vomica, Sepia*
Occipital extending to eyes and forehead	*Belladonna, Gelsemium, Lachesis, Silicea*
to above right eye	*Pulsatilla*
to above left eye	*Sepia*
Right sided	*Belladonna, Bryonia, Pulsatilla*
Left sided	*Lachesis, Phosphorus, Sepia*
Vertex	*Arsenicum, Gelsemium, Lachesis, Nux vomica, Pulsatilla, Sepia, Sulphur*

Some Sensations

Boring	*Belladonna, Hepar sulphuris, Sepia*
Bruised pain	*Arnica, Gelsemium, Ignatia, Lycopodium, Nux vomica*
Burning pain	*Rhus toxicodendron, Silicea Apis, Arnica, Arsenicum, Belladonna, Lachesis Lycopodium, Phosphorus, Silicea, Sulphur*
Burning pain on the vertex	*Sulphur*
Bursting pain	*Belladonna, Bryonia, Calcarea carbonica, Lachesis*
Constrictive – like a tight band	*Aconite, Gelsemium, Mercurius, Natrum muriaticum, Sulphur*
As if crushed	*Ignatia, Lachesis, Phosphorus, Sepia, Silicea*
Like a thousand hammers	*Natrum muriaticum*
Red hot needles from one temple to the other	*Arsenicum (right to left)*
As if a nail were driven into the forehead	*Ignatia, Thuja*
As if from the root of the nose	*Ipecacuanha*
Throbbing pain	*Aconite, Belladonna, Bryonia, Gelsemium, Hypericum, Lachesis, Lycopodium, Natrum muriaticum, Pulsatilla, Sepia, Silicea*
Like a weight on the vertex	*Nux vomica*

Remedies

Nux vomica

This is a remedy of the tension headache, and the bilious headache, and the migraine. How can it cover so much?

The personality of this type predisposes to the headache. They are perfectionists and workaholics. The essence of the remedy is *'out of harmony'*. This theme runs throughout the remedy's symptoms and is especially found in its modalities and exciting causes. They have a sense of order and correctness so we label them *fastidious*. In another time we might have said they were righteous. They are **impulsive**. The impetus of the remedy is action so the most powerful exciting cause is a block to action leading to *frustration*. They have a great deal of drive, doing too much.

Ultimately this exhausts their nerves so we get the migraine but first we get *impatience* and *intolerance*. They cannot wait in queues – what a waste of time. They rev up their car at traffic lights or drum their fingers needing to move or act. Tension and spasm builds up in the muscles especially of the shoulders where they carry such an enormous load. This is where the *tension* headache comes in. The muscles are held so tight there is no flow. The muscles knot up. Pain results. It is a gnawing pain.

They are like a coiled spring ready to leap on any defaulter. Their anger is explosive. Heat and tension in the head draws the brows together in a frown. Arterial hypertension may lead to high blood pressure, even to *apoplexy*, when they *blow their top*. To lower the tension they indulge – coffee, alcohol, cigarettes. They will rattle their worry beads. They will develop habits to keep on the move – scratching their head, their beard, their ear, tapping their foot. They may lash out or feel murderous towards anyone in their way. They can be terrible bullies, harassing others to do their part, or do what the *Nux vomica* patient sees as needed.

In leisure they indulge their senses. This could be fast cars or sex but in our society most commonly they eat – the new restaurant, the new dish, the best wine or finest brandy. They overeat, preferring *stimulating foods* that are rich in sauces, or fats, or spices, etc. They crave strongly seasoned foods. This is one of our most common liver remedies. Out of harmony becomes nausea but so intense is the spasm in the gut that there is reversed peristalsis so they say *'if only I could be sick'*. Indeed, if they vomit they are fine. They are worse for heat that creates more activity in the abdomen but better for stimulating fresh air. Fresh air feels clean to them.

More indulgence creates a sluggish liver so their most common symptom is *constipation*. With liver congestion they are irritable, cursing violently at trifling incidents or the door that gets in the way. Their frown may become permanent lines between the eyes, *liver lines*. The dull head may feel heavy, *as if there is a weight on their vertex*. The head is pulled down between the shoulder in a typical stance, as if to avoid the load on top of the head. Now we may see the start of nerve strain in the sense organs which are over-sensitive. Their eyes are sensitive to the light. Most particular they are *sensitive to noise* especially to music that has a rhythm and beat which may not be their harmony. The slightest noise, the rustle at the other end of the railway carriage, the whiny pitch of the personal stereo, drives them insane with rage. Be careful they are *quarrelsome* and *do not tolerate contradiction*.

Eventually they are nervously exhausted. They may shake and tremble with exhaustion. They cannot rest or relax. They cannot sleep. The agitation continues. Here I find music does help them to sleep because with no other stimulus they can let themselves go into its rhythm. In extreme cases they may be dizzy and nauseous. The migraine headache is one sided, right, with sensitivity to light, to foods such as cheese that are difficult to digest. There may be relief from firm pressure because by now they have lost any point from which to balance. They feel strained and out of it. Yet rest is anathema. Send them to occupations like the garden or to walk to give them recreational movement that is creative and calming.

> **EXERCISE**
>
> From the symptom picture of the remedy above, can you pick out symptoms of:
> - Time
> - Location
> - Sensation
> - Modality
> - Intensity?
>
> Which are the concomitant symptoms?
>
> Which are the: a) exciting causes?
>
> b) maintaining causes?

Pulsatilla

This is a very different remedy from *Nux vomica*. As a sycotic remedy it works through the lymphatic system and mucus membrane. It has a profound affect on fluid balance and flow throughout the body. Thus it is a remedy of the sinus headache or the sluggish congestive constitution that is subject to Premenstrual Syndrome.

The body tissues of the *Pulsatilla* patient are relaxed. The character is *mild* and *yielding, affectionate* and *desiring to please*. Symptoms arise when they are cut off from others through *grief, disappointed love* and *loss*. These exciting causes may be activated less intensely when loss is after arguments, being ignored or embarrassed in any way that isolates them. They may *burst into tears* or *sulk* solemnly. They are often described as cuddly, or wet.

When *exposed to cold and wet*, especially wet feet, they develop colds. The mucus membrane lining the upper respiratory tract produces copious mucus. The tonsils on the right side may be inflamed and throb. Even the cervical glands may be involved. As the cold progresses, every possible part secretes. The right ear may become congested with catarrh and throb painfully – this is the involvement of the minor organ we will talk about in Lesson 5. *Pulsatilla* only ever produces a low grade fever. It is more likely that the catarrh will spread so the sinus in the head may be congested – a true head cold. *Throbbing pains* occur in congested parts.

The modalities at this stage are interesting in showing the difference between the modalities of a part and the general modalities. *Pulsatilla* is generally *better for continued motion* that stimulates the relaxed part so encouraging flow and avoiding stagnancy. Locally this may be seen as *worse lying down* when the head becomes full of mucus because there is no drainage. When they lie on one side the mucus flows to block that nostril. In the morning they are markedly worse re catarrh because it has not been able to drain in the night. Locally they may easily become dizzy or even faint as they stand up quickly. The ears may ring as flow starts in the ears. The throbbing may be violent as the catarrh drains from the sinus. The worsening locally can be seen in this context to be the initial aggravation, the long term effect being amelioration.

In the next stage the catarrh thickens then dries. The symptom picture in the dry stage is one of stuffiness much relieved by *fresh air*. The local heat that got things moving above now becomes an aggravation when the *Pulsatilla* patient at this stage is much much *worse for heat* that further dries the mucus membrane. So modalities can also indicate the stage of development of the symptom picture. This change in emphasis of the modality also explains the seeming contradiction that some of the books may say 'better from ...' whilst others say 'worse from ...' or it may explain the confusion of those new to Homoeopathy when the book says 'better from ... **and** worse from ...'. In a remedy like *Pulsatilla* this may be just a little bit easier because the colour of the catarrh changes as the disease deepens so it may start clear then become white and end up yellow or even green.

The symptoms above can be explained by Anatomy and Physiology and the type of constitution. Other symptoms characteristic of *Pulsatilla* show its Individuality. The headache of *Pulsatilla* locates characteristically in the *occiput moving over to above the right eye*. A keynote symptom is *wandering pains* that flit from place to place. Thus the throbbing pains in the sinus headache may move about all over the place giving quite a vague presentation from the patient until you realise that is what is happening. It can be equally confusing when you go to give sympathy to an aged aunt with rheumatism – as if she has lost her marbles, how can it move about?

The key is the relaxed state of the tissue and the fact that catarrh either flows or dryness rebounds along to another part. Whilst this may be easily explained in tubes and ducts, Homoeopathy defies anatomical explanation at times, so luckily we need only describe the symptom as clearly as possible and correlate it with a similar symptom produced in the provings, such symptoms as Strange, Rare and Peculiar.

Where the system is more deeply affected, we will find the aggravation *worse before menstruation* or even *worse puberty* or *worse after pregnancy*, or *worse menopause*. *Pulsatilla* has a profound effect on the female reproductive cycle. Often the period is late. At menarche the onset of menstruation may be delayed even until 17 years. Being such an emotional remedy we often find it when the periods have stopped, *amenorrhoea*, because of grief or after losing the first boyfriend. Because flow is sluggish, the period may be heavy and clotted and even painful.

Some of the worst cases I have seen of dysmenorrhoea are in young girls with a sluggish venous flow. Later this will be evidenced also as varicose veins. The local modality is *better heat* as a hot water bottle that increases the flow. This is not applicable in the varicose vein even though it may help because here there may be a complication of clots as phlebitis.

Sluggish venous flow is evident in the digestive symptoms where there is difficulty absorbing rich foods. Pork and fat are especially difficult. There is a link between the lymphatic system that produces the mucus to mucus membrane and the lymph vessels in the villae of the small intestines that absorb fat. It is this relationship that produces the puppy fat of the podgy young *Pulsatilla* or in failing to produce it in the immature young girl offsets the menarche. Later the matron will struggle in vain with chubbiness. This may not be helped by the fact that the *Pulsatilla* patient has a preference for rich food in the form of *cream cakes, ice cream* and *butter* or *pastries usually rich in cream and butter*.

Portal vein stasis arises giving symptoms similar to *Nux vomica* which is a useful acute in the *Pulsatilla* patient – nausea, constipation, headache of a bilious type. Like *Nux vomica* the *Pulsatilla* patient may also have haemorrhoids that easily bleed. The difference between the two remedies is tension. *Nux vomica* is hard, whereas *Pulsatilla* is soft, e.g. in the abdomen, in manner and temperament.

This same laxity of tissue makes them very susceptible to *tobacco smoke* which attacks the mucus membrane by first stimulating then paralysing the little cilia (hairs) that sweep the respiratory system clear with their rhythmic beating. At a deeper level it attacks smooth and visceral muscles so the small intestine and veins are susceptible, hence why smokers often suffer from vein problems.

Later in life the catarrhal state of *Pulsatilla* is found in rheumatism that is *better for continued gentle motion, better local heat, is worse on the right side, has pains that flit from joint to joint, and is worse getting soaked*. Note how all the modalities we have learned above now fit into a full symptoms picture. All we now need to add to get the constitutional type is the temperament of *yielding, pleasing, desires company* and *weepy*, or *sulky*. If we can add the points of change or exciting causes (< *grief, disappointed love, loss*) we have a very clear situation in which *Pulsatilla* is the curative remedy.

Whatever the age, Pulsatilla patients can be expected at the start of the year when the seasons start to warm up. This is the Hay Fever time. Colds start with April showers. Later in the year they have headaches with the sun. Into the Autumn there is an influx when the central heating goes on in the office or school. According to the stage they will come in with catarrh and colds, or headaches. The rheumatism will start with the cold weather or if they get soaked. A keynote is *getting the feet wet*.

> **EXERCISE**
>
> From the symptom picture of the remedy above, can you pick out symptoms of: Time
>
> Location
>
> Sensation
>
> Modality?
>
> Which are the concomitant symptoms?
>
> Are there any Strange, Rare and Peculiar symptoms?
>
> Which are the: a) exciting causes?
>
> b) maintaining causes?

Bryonia

Characteristically, this is a very similar remedy to *Pulsatilla* since it acts on mucus membrane lining tissue to produce *first copious mucus then dryness*. It is also *right sided*. As in *Pulsatilla* the cold will move into the glands, especially the tonsils, or into the sinus as a head cold or into the minor organ, the right ear. Unlike *Pulsatilla*, *Bryonia* then affects the chest as bronchitis or even deeper as pleurisy or pneumonia. It affects the liver rather than the kidneys so it is a remedy of the *bilious* headache. It is a remedy of congestion when that is due to a sluggish liver. This is a very different kind of congestion from the lymphatic kind of *Pulsatilla*. This is a different constitutional type where *constitution* refers to the underlying weaknesses giving rise to different types of acutes or different symptoms. So like *Pulsatilla*, we can say the metabolism of *Bryonia* is 'slow in onset' showing less vitality than an inflammatory remedy like *Belladonna*. Thus the acutes that arise will only have low grade fevers and, as the disease penetrates deeper through the body's defences than *Belladonna*, it is the lymphatic system and the glands that are affected producing what the doctor might call *'an infection'* – coloured catarrh..

White Bryony is wild hops. Its action is *soporific*, slowing down metabolism as when too much beer is drunk it causes sluggish liver. In a really congestive state, the *Bryonia* patient resembles the drunkard with a dull red face and fuzzy head, or dulled consciousness, who is touchy and irritable when roused to action. Whilst you will see the dulled, slow consciousness and irritability, the patient will be really ill before you will see this dull red face, i.e. may have bronchitis.

White Bryony grows in hedgerows where it clings to other plants for support. Its greatest sensitivity is to damp conditions so it is no surprise that constitutionally the *Bryonia* patient is susceptible to *cold, wet conditions*. Lung problems do not fare well in damp basements. After being soaked, inflammation may set in so the glands on the right side are enlarged. Copious mucus is produced from engorged, dull red mucus membrane – see where the colour comes in locally! Catarrh that is white at the start will turn *yellow* where *Pulsatilla* will turn green. The more engorged the mucus membrane then the greater the *throbbing pains*. As the *dryness* sets in there will be increased *sensitivity to heat* and the pain will change to *stitching*, < *movement*. Indeed two keynotes appear here that will distinguish *Bryonia* from *Pulsatilla* – the stitching pain will be described as *sticking*, and there will be *a great thirst*.

The art of Homoeopathy is often in picking up the intensity of a symptom. In *Bryonia* there is a great thirst – the patient will drink bucketsful, or gallons. Now this is an exaggeration but it points to something very unusual, a whole glassful at one gulp or more than one glassful, perhaps. *Pulsatilla* is notably thirstless but today I have seen this symptom hidden by the fact they comfort drink sweet drinks or hot drinks, as they comfort eat. *Pulsatilla* does not drink because they are thirsty. The thirst of the *Bryonia* patient is unquenchable. Exaggeration is also seen in the *bursting pains* or the *explosive* headache which is very different from the fullness and stuffiness of engorgement in *Pulsatilla*.

The *Bryonia* patient appears *dopey*. Whereas *Pulsatilla* will whine, *Bryonia moans*. They *want to go home* or will *worry about work* and/or their financial security. Like the plant, the *Bryonia* patient is *insecure*. This constitutional thread becomes visible in the personality when it makes them cautious and careful. You will find them in secure jobs with good prospects or pension. There will be a clear routine or procedure. They are good accountants or form the bulwark of the firm as middle managers. The irritation will then arise when they are stretched or under pressure of a deadline. The effect on the constitution may cause an acute – their digestion may be upset or if vitality is really lowered they will be prone to chesty colds.

As in *Nux vomica*, the *Bryonia* patient is sensuous so they *overindulge*, putting pressure on the liver which creates or increases the congestion. This is where the headache comes in as an acute. It is *worse before menstruation,* or *worse after alcohol.* The sensation is fullness becoming *bursting*, < movement, < heat. Central heating is intolerable. They are worse after exertion or eating which increases activity of circulation or causes heating. Of course you will see the irritability now and if menopausal you may see the flushed dull red face. They are *worse stooping* which increases congestion to the head. So the *Bryonia* patient with a headache is to be found lying perfectly still, moving only to quaff large draughts of water, and they are extremely irritable if disturbed in any way. In this last symptom, the *Bryonia* patient can resemble the *Nux vomica* patient.

Where the constitution is weakened and digestion is very poor they may vomit bile with the headache. More commonly they will be constipated, < before menstruation. The stool will be dry and hard. In the worst cases the stool may even appear burnt.

As a remedy of glands, as well as tonsillitis, it commonly affects the breasts so we may find sore breasts before menstruation or it can be found useful in mastitis where the symptoms agree, i.e. right sided, *stone hard.* As a glandular remedy it is frequently specific in mumps when this is right sided. As well as the parotid glands, the breasts, the testes or the ovaries may be affected because there is a constitutional weakness.

The other common ailment where we find this remedy is in coughs. It is a major component of many proprietary cough mixtures. The main symptoms of the cough are that it starts after a soaking or exposure to dampness and is *worse inspiration.* Each time they cough you will see them grasp the throat or the chest to prevent the pain caused by movement. The headache is greatly increased with coughing. The cough comes with colds and flus. We will discuss this in a later lesson where we will want to compare it with other remedies.

> **EXERCISE**
>
> From the symptoms above can you pick out the following:
> Time
> Location
> Sensation
> Modality?
>
> What is the concomitant symptom to the headache?
>
> What are the: a) exciting causes?
> b) maintaining causes?
>
> I have mentioned mastitis and mumps above. Can you apply the characteristic symptoms of *Bryonia* to describe the patient's case more fully?

If you can do these exercises after the remedies in this lesson, you will be well on the way to thinking homoeopathically.

Repertorising

Since there are well over 2000 homoeopathic remedies, the question of memory must arise. How is it possible to remember every symptom of every remedy, especially when symptoms have different values? The answer is that Homoeopaths have constructed **repertories**, the most famous of which is Kent's, now over 100 years old. Of course it has been updated and added to since it was first constructed.

A repertory contains all the symptoms that have been discovered by Homoeopaths whilst doing provings on remedies. Remember, during the proving of a remedy, healthy individuals now called **provers** take the remedy until they produce symptoms. This is based on the homeopathic principle that all medicines have two actions, the first being opposite to the second. So, if you keep taking a medicine you will get to its second action. If you are ill when you take that medicine the first action will make you worse but the second action will remove the symptoms. If you have no illness when you take a homoeopathic remedy then it will make you ill by producing symptoms according to its symptom picture. This is the proving that tells the Homoeopath the field of action of the medicine. Thus over the 200 years of modern Homoeopathy, there is little that is not known about many remedies, which means Homoeopathy can be very accurate.

The symptoms produced during a proving are entered into the Repertory in three grades thus:

- **Bold** type when everyone produced that symptom so it is seen as characteristic of the remedy
- *Italic* type when a large group of provers produced that symptom so it is commonly associated with the remedy
- Ordinary type when only a few provers produced that symptom.

The last is deceptive as, on a bell-shaped curve, the lesser symptoms at one end of the curve may correspond to provers who had little resonance to the remedy whilst at the other end provers very sensitive to the remedy may produce keynotes of the remedy. In any one proving, provers will have varying degrees of resonance to the remedy proved so will respond with different degrees to the remedy. Thus the Homoeopath will find the repertory an invaluable aid to memory but a limited tool as such provings may produce only a statistical average of the reaction to the remedy. More recent provings recognise this weakness and have tried to correct it, as has various editing of the repertory since its inception.

The process of repertorising draws together all the symptoms of the patient then trawls through the repertory to find which remedies have these symptoms. A good Homoeopath achieves accuracy by using only those symptoms of Individuality and Susceptibility. Also, just as the entries have different values, the Homeopath has a hierarchy of value so that Strange, Rare and Peculiar symptoms (which point to individuality) are at the top of the hierarchy, followed by Mental and Emotional symptoms, then General symptoms (which denote metabolic changes, or the whole) and finally Particular symptoms of the parts that compose the whole. Common symptoms have little role in prescribing a homoeopathic remedy because they do not allow us to discriminate precisely and accurately. However, it would be false to say they have no value as they can determine the disease pattern and therefore prognosis of the illness. They simply do not help to find the remedy.

At the end of the next few lessons, I have constructed summary tables that you can look up like a repertory to help you prescribe more accurately. You should also study the *materia medica* of the remedy to ensure it is a good fit. Remember the Law of Similars is **like cures like**.

SHORT REPERTORY OF HEADACHES

NEURALGIC

Occurs	LEFT side	acon, arn, *bry,* gels, hep, ign, **lach,** *merc,* **sep,** *sil*
	RIGHT side	*acon, arn,* **ars, bell, bry,** *hep, ign,* merc, **nux v, puls,** *sil*
	Over LEFT EYE	acon, arn, *ars,* **bry,** *ign,* lach, nux v, pils, *sep*
	Then right	*lach*
	Over RIGHT EYE	acon, ars, *bell,* bry, *gels, ign,* lach, *nat m,* rhus t,
	Then left	*nat m,* sep
< light		arn, *ars,* **bell,** *gels, ign, nat m,* nux v, *sep, sil*
< *artificial light*		**sep,** *sil*
< noise		acon, arn, *ars,* **bell,** *bry,* gels, ign, *lach,* nux v, sil
drops things		bell, bry, *lach, nat m,* nux v, sep
forgets words		*arn,* lach, *nat m,* nux v, puls
mistakes in (using wrong) words		*arn,* hep, sep
speech incoherent		ars, *bell,* **bry,** *gels,* hep, **lach,** merc, **rhus t**

TENSION

Sidedness as above

Occiput	*acon,* **arn,** *ars,* **bell, bry, cimic,** coloc, **gels,** hep, *ign, lach,* led, merc, nat m, **nux v,** *puls, rhus t,* **sep, sil**
Extending above eyes	gels, **lach,** *sep, sil*
Down back of neck	bell, *bry, hep,* merc, **nux v,** sep
Pain — Throbbing	**bell,** *gels,* ign, **lach,** *led, nat m,* puls, *sep*
Hammering	*nat m*
As of a band	*gels,* merc
< stooping	acon, *gels*
< mental exertion	*cimic, gels,* ign, rhus t

BILIOUS

Sidedness as above
Throbbing as above

Heavy weight on the vertex	*ars,* **bell, lach,** *led,* **nux v,** *rhus t,* **sil**
As if would burst	ars, **bell, bry,** *hep,* ign, **lach, merc, nat m,** *puls,* rhus t, **sep,** *sil*
< lying down	ars, *bell, coloc, gels,* hep, ign, led, *merc,* puls, *rhus t,* sep
< heat	acon, *arn,* **ars,** *bell,* bry, coloc, *hep, ign, lach,* **nat m,** nux v, puls, rhus t, l*sep,* **sil**
< rich food	*bry,* **puls,** *sep*
< *cheese*	*ars, bry,* coloc, *rhus t*
< *fatty food*	acon, *ars,* bell, bry, hep, merc, nat m, nux v, **puls,** *sep,* sil
with nausea	acon, arn, *ars, bry, coloc,* gels, hep, ign, *lach, merc,* nat m, nux v, puls, rhus t, *sep,* sil
nausea < smell of food	*ars, sep*
Vision, black spots	acon, arn, *bell, cimic, gels,*merc, **nat m,** nux v, *rhus t,* **sep, sil**

SINUS

Frontal	**acon, arn, ars, bell, bry,** cimic, *coloc,* gels, **hep, ign,** *lach,* led, **merc, nat m, nux v, puls,** *sep,* **sil**
Over eyes	acon, *arn, ars, bell, bry, gels,* hep, ign, *lach,* merc, *nat m,* **puls,** *sep,* **sil**
Behind eyes	acon, gels, lach, led, rhus t, sep
Feels full/stuffy	*acon,* arn, ars, *bell,* **bry,** *coloc, gels,* hep, lach, merc, *nat m,* nux v, puls, *rhus t,* sep, **sil**
< stooping	acon, arn, **bell, bry,** *coloc, gels, hep,* ign, **merc,** *nat m,* nux v, **puls,** *sil*
< lying down	bry, coloc, *gels,* merc
< turning the head suddenly	gels, ign, *nat m*
< heat	sep
> open air	acon, coloc, lach, merc, *nux v, puls,* sep

READING

Fritjof Kapra   The Turning Point   Harper Collins

> *This is a book by a modern physicist who challenges our mode of thought – in this book especially in relation to healing. Other books include* The Tao of Physics *and* The Web of Life.

THOUGHTS TO PONDER

> *It is the morbidly affected vital force alone that produces diseases, so that the morbid phenomena (symptoms) perceptible to our senses express at the same time all the internal change, that is to say, the whole morbid derangement of the internal dynamis; in a word, they (the symptoms) reveal the whole disease; also, the disappearance under treatment of all the morbid phenomena (symptoms) ... necessarily implies the restoration of the integrity of the vital force and, therefore, the recovered health of the whole organism.*
>
> Para 12, The Organon of the Rational Art of Healing
> Samuel Hahnemann

> *Therefore disease ... considered as a thing separate from the living whole, from the organism and its animating vital force, and hidden in the interior, be it of ever so subtle a character, is an absurdity, that could only be imagined by minds of a materialistic stamp, and has for thousands of years given to the prevailing system of medicine all those pernicious impulses that have made it a truly mischievous (non-healing) art.*
>
> Para 13, The Organon of the Rational Art of Healing
> Samuel Hahnemann

LESSON 4   Sore Throats

Aims: To discuss the homoeopathic treatment of sore throats.
To show how symptoms build up into a symptom picture.
To demonstrate different levels of defence response.
To show the relationship of symptoms to Anatomy and Physiology.
To discuss the role of Individuality and Susceptibility.
To demonstrate how the Total Symptom Picture represents the action of the Vital Force.
To study *Belladonna* and *Lachesis*.

Keywords used:
Defence system
systemic response
exciting cause
inflammation
suppuration
Strange, Rare and Peculiar symptoms

inner tube
congestion
Individuality
Susceptibility
Total Symptom Picture

What is a Sore Throat?

This common ailment is associated with 'colds' which involve systemic response such as fever, drowsiness, and chill. In some people there will be no systemic response but only local symptoms such as glandular swellings, runny nose, etc.

In the healthiest individuals (i.e. *Belladonna* and *Aconite* types), local symptoms may be inflammation of the local lining of the Upper Respiratory system, e.g. epithelial tissue of the pharynx area, giving heat, redness, swelling and throbbing pains. These are the common symptoms of inflammation. When produced after exposure to the exciting cause, *cold conditions* as in the case of *Belladonna* and *Aconite*, the symptom becomes more individual. Individuality leads us to differentiate one homoeopathic remedy from another, e.g. *Belladonna* is right sided, *Aconite* is left sided; *Belladonna* is < wet cold, *Aconite* is < dry cold.

Inflammation is the first line of defence occurring when there is increased flow of blood to an area. The type of pain may depend on the structure at that location. In inflammation pain is usually of a *throbbing* nature but it may be *burning* as the part heats up, or *shooting* as spasm is involved. In *Aconite* there is often *tearing* pain showing the involvement of nerves. The effect on nerves is part of the Individuality, uniqueness, of *Aconite*. Where mast cells are involved in inflammation there may be oedema or, more commonly, itching, the symptom of the Individuality of *Hepar sulphuris* or *Rhus toxicodendron*. In remedies such as *Apis mellifica* the characteristic pattern of the remedy is to produce oedema. There may be so much oedema that the patient has other symptoms such as the throat closing – < *swallowing*. Where the part is very dry there may be *stick-like* sensations individual to six remedies that include *Hepar sulphuris, Nitric Acidum,* and *Silica*. Where spasm occurs in connective tissue there may be Strange, Rare and Peculiar symptoms, as in *Cantharis,* where even the thought of drinking water produces the spasm – a truly individual symptom.

The next stage of the defence system is suppuration [1] when the specialised lining cells of the inner tube secrete mucus that thickens to catarrh as white blood cells are involved.[2] This condition is often labelled infectious [3] especially when the catarrh turns green or yellow. The thickening tells us that the seriousness

---
[1] My label and I am not 100% happy with it. Help!!!
[2] I get quite uptight about people who suppress temperature with substances such as paracetamol. Apart from its action on the liver hindering the detox programme, the organism needs that high temperature as certain defence mechanisms only function in high temperature. Intervention is needed only when there is a problem. Likewise, I was fascinated to discover that that wonderful body in producing excess lubrication aids the action of the macrophages (the big boys of the immune system) that can move only by creeping along wet surfaces. Thanks for that information Lindsay Campbell.
[3] Check back to 'contagious' acutes in the Introduction.

of the disturbance is increasing or, when the patient goes to this stage immediately, that the patient is less healthy in general. From the speedy reaction of the blood in inflammation, we now have the slow seepage from the lymph system, the great sea of the body. The white blood cells carry the immune response in the T leucocytes. The phagocyte type of white blood cell engulfs the toxins and foreign matter to produce pus.

Excess secretions contain these defenders that we now see as *pus* or *catarrh*. Greater disturbance is localised to the lymph glands, especially the tonsils in throat problems. These may become swollen and inflamed. Since toxins are produced, it is just one step to generalised ill feeling with dullness, sleepiness, general aches, overheating or chill. These may be *common* symptoms of colds or flu. The pain produced at this stage may not be so intense. It is often described as a dull ache, or soreness. If throbbing, it is a dull throb. The main sensation is of congestion, fullness. There may be problems swallowing because of this congestion. When the catarrh starts to dry up there will be stitching pain that often extends to the ear on swallowing, e.g. in *Bryonia, Mercurius, Lachesis*. This is more individual. The Individuality of a remedy may be indicated when the tonsils are affected always on the right side, or the left, or if the pain moves from right to left, *Pulsatilla, Lycopodium,* or from left to right, *Lachesis, Silica.* In severe cases the glands may harden, *Silica, Calcarea, Graphites*. Where sepsis exists, we often speak of a quinsy throat. Where the throat, tonsils or fauces are ulcerated and the breath foul, the remedies indicated may include *Lachesis, Mercurius,* and *Baptisia*.

The exact location involved gives the specific name to the sore throat, e.g. laryngitis, pharyngitis, tonsillitis.

When the voice is overused, the connective tissue of the vocal cords is strained. This is laryngitis. The swelling of these ligaments causes a characteristic husky voice. Usually there is also excessive catarrh as the lining epithelial cells secrete excessively to protect the structures. The homoeopathic remedy required must include in its Individuality an ability to act on connective tissue, e.g. *Rhus toxicodendron, Causticum.* These could then be differentiated by Individuality from those remedies where the huskiness will come from excessive catarrh, e.g. *Phosphorus, Lachesis, Argentum nitricum.*

I hope this helps you to see how precisely we look at symptoms homoeopathically. We are looking for what is unusual, what stops and makes us hesitate, what is Individual in the symptom picture. To do this we do not ignore Medical Sciences. Indeed we need to know the *Common* symptoms thoroughly in order to determine what is individual or Strange, Rare and Peculiar.

EXERCISE

Review the Anatomy and Physiology in a suitable textbook.

Draw a diagram clearing labelling: The Adenoids
Tonsils
Larynx
Pharynx

Where are the vocal cords?

Philosophy

Now we have learned at little of how the Homoeopath looks at symptoms in a sore throat, it is relevant to look more closely at the mechanism of Homoeopathy that puts this information together to find the *Similimum,* the appropriate remedy.

Individuality

Put very simply the Law of Similars is about matching two symptom pictures, that of the patient and that of the remedy. The degree of similarity is the degree of resonance that determines the efficiency of the remedy. So how do we determine similarity?

Since Hahnemann's day we have put greatest value on the symptom that is most representative of Individuality and uniqueness. So in our hierarchy of symptoms, *Strange, Rare and Peculiar* symptoms come at the top, then *Mental and Emotional* symptoms that express personality and temperament, then *General* symptoms that represent the constitution and metabolism.

We also put greater value on a *full symptom* that has Time, Location, Sensation and Modality. Two or more of these attributes make a symptom more unique and individual. J. T. Kent says a *prescribing symptom* is something that stops and makes us hesitate because it is not common but unique or individual to that person. To match a remedy at this degree of uniqueness is to get a truly individual match.

Susceptibility

The *Exciting Cause* comes very high up the hierarchy of values. Indeed in acute cases it is at the top because this is the *point of change* representing a reaction of the Vital Force to something to which it is *susceptible*. It is also Time.

Individuality and Susceptibility are the key to success in homoeopathic prescribing. Individuality enables a good match in the symptom picture but there is more to resonance than mere description. The Vital Force is an energy. In other words, it is dynamic and responsive. When Individuality is extended to cover that to which the Vital Force is most reactive, i.e. its Susceptibility, there is a match to the dynamic energy at the core of the Vital Force. Susceptibility is indicated most clearly in three ways:

- *The exciting cause* of the acute symptom picture is the point at which the Vital Force was newly disturbed.

- *The point of change* of the chronic symptom picture may arise from an exciting cause to produce an acute symptom picture, or it may be a maintaining cause, or a failure to recover from an acute illness that produces a deeper level of the disease process.

- *The modality* may be most important in the chronic case as it is the edge of the pattern, the containing factor that shows the stress lines, or weaknesses, of the organism.

Susceptibility can be seen as the weakness of the Vital Force or that to which it resonates.

Precision, Clarity and Accuracy

George Vithoulkas talks of *precision, clarity* and *accuracy* referring to the quality of the data obtained in case taking. How precisely have we described the symptom? If the symptom is abdominal pain exactly where in the abdomen is it? Exactly how would we describe the pain? How clear is the meaning we have derived from the information? How accurately have we represented the case? The more precise we are about the symptoms then the more accurate the match to the remedy. The more individual and unique the symptom, the greater is the clarity of the symptom picture and the more accurate the match of the remedy to the Vital Force.

Total Symptom Picture

Of equal importance to how the symptom picture breaks down is how it is put together – the Total Symptom Picture. All symptoms are produced by the Vital Force yet we know little of the Vital Force because it is intangible and invisible, like electricity and magnetism. We see only the results of its activity

– the symptoms. They are the only way we can 'see' what the Vital Force is up to and how we can help it. Therefore the pattern of symptoms is very important to us. When disturbed by an Exciting Cause, the Vital Force produces a group of symptoms – *a symptom picture*. Every symptom produced is related if only by time. When we match this pattern of symptoms to that of a remedy we match the Total Symptom Picture – *all* the symptoms.

The Vital Force holds the totality of our being. It is in touch with all. The nearest we can come to see how it acts in every second of our existence is through homeostatic balance when our temperature, heart beat, blood pressure, breathing, etc is regulated. The Vital Force acts on the whole. Homoeopathy is holistic because it acts on the Vital Force. This should explain why the Homoeopath relates all symptoms to the whole. Even if the problem is *only* sore throats the Homoeopath will take the time to look at the overall health picture to find out where the sore throats fit in.

Putting it all together

Whilst the Vital Force may localise a symptom it will never produce that symptom in isolation. Thus when we look at sore throats we may choose a different remedy depending on the temperament, or Mental and Emotional symptoms, of the patient. The mildness of *Pulsatilla*, the fearfulness of *Aconite*, the suspicion of *Lachesis* or the rage of *Belladonna* become important differentiating symptoms. They express the Individuality of the remedy. In the last lesson we saw how the constitution has weaknesses that predispose it to produce certain types of symptoms; hence *Belladonna* acts on the blood but produces a different kind of congestion from *Lachesis* that also acts on the blood to produce congestion because of its slowness and tendency to coagulate. On the *General* level the congestion of *Belladonna* is due to inflammation so has heat and fullness with shooting pains and bright redness, even delirium, showing the activity of the blood. *Lachesis*, on the other hand, has heat and fullness with a constricting pain, dull redness, dullness of consciousness and the bloody discharge and smell of sepsis. We spoke in the last lesson of *Pulsatilla* as a congestive remedy. The congestion of *Pulsatilla* is catarrhal. On the general level it produces bland catarrh, usually white going towards green as the situation deepens. The pain is a dull ache. The suppuration goes towards a dryness that is stuffy whereas the dryness of *Belladonna* is produced by the intense heat of inflammation.

When we match the remedy, we match the Total Symptom Picture, *all* the symptoms of the patient to those of a remedy. It is the Vital Force that is disturbed. The type and level of symptom tells us how deeply it is disturbed. The more disturbed, then the more Mental and Emotional and General symptoms. The healthier the Vital Force, the more able it is to localise the disturbance to local symptoms, Particulars, and the faster it will produce the symptom picture.

Hence in the sore throat we decide first whether it is local, as in overuse of the voice where there is a maintaining cause, or just one symptom of a 'cold' that is an acute illness with an exciting cause, or part of a chronic picture of debility when it is not the sore throat but the lowered vitality we need to treat. The Homoeopath treats each of these differently.

> **EXERCISE**
>
> It would be useful to collect some symptom pictures of sore throats then decide which of the above categories they fit into.

Remedies for Sore Throats

Note that the Individuality is printed below in *italics*. Also, I have put in the defence mechanism and Location or affinity of the remedy's action which may help with accurate selection of the remedy and its potency as it tells us about vitality.

Aconite produces heat, redness, dryness and swelling that gives rise to *choking*. This occurs usually *after exposure to cold*. Often it is the tonsils that are affected and swell. As usual with *Aconite* there will be *intense pain, restlessness and anxiety*. There may be *a thirst for cold drinks*. This is related to the acute throat as inflammation is temporarily > coldness but it is also a general characteristic of *Aconite*.

Aconite is also a remedy of croup after exposure to dry cold conditions. Usually there is fever and the child *grasps the throat on each spasm* that produces a *hoarse dry cough*.

INFLAMMATION – EPITHELIAL *of the lining tissue, plus, sometimes the tonsils, LYMPH GLANDS. Left sided. DRYNESS.*

Belladonna may produce a dry, hot, red throat as in *Aconite* but on *exposure to wet, cold conditions*. The *right tonsil* is usually affected becoming so swollen the patient *swallows constantly* even when this chokes them. They can swallow little food or drink. To gain relief they *bend the head backwards* because this gives more room to the swollen tonsils. The pain is *throbbing* and there is much *sensitivity to touch*. Often there is so much fever that one patient described it as if *being so hot the clothes are heated up*.

INFLAMMATION – EPITHELIAL *of the lining tissue, sometimes the tonsils, LYMPH GLANDS. Right sided. DRYNESS.*

Bryonia The cause is usually *exposure to damp*. Here vitality is lower than that in *Aconite* and *Belladonna* so the patient is slower to produce the symptoms after exposure: 24-48 hours. Soon the throat will be stuffed up with much catarrh that starts white and may become *yellow* and *tenacious as it dries up*. The throat becomes *very dry*. They *crave much water* but the throat is so swollen that each swallowing movement produces the characteristic *stitching pain*. They clasp the throat to stop the movement. It may be the *right tonsil* or the back of the throat that is swollen. The red colour is a much duller hue than the above two remedies. The patient is *irritable* and *adverse to heat and touch*.

INFLAMMATION –> SUPPURATIVE – EPITHELIAL *with catarrh moving to dryness. LYMPH GLANDS. It is more glandular. Right sided.*

Hepar sulphuris *affects the glands*. You will notice this in the tonsils and cervical glands, *right sided*. The glands swell and harden after *exposure to cold conditions*. Suppuration sets in rapidly so the *breath is foul – sour*. It is a remedy of the *quinsy* throat. At first there is much *yellow mucus* which they *hawk up continually*, then the mucus membrane dries up giving the characteristic *sensation of a stick* in the dry throat as the sides touch. They may feel a *plug* from a lump of tenacious mucus that will not hawk up. As they yawn or swallow *a stitching pain stretches to the right ear*. They are so prone to suppuration that these sore throats are recurrent.

Since this remedy affects connective tissue the voice may be *hoarse*, or even *lost*. There is a hard dry cough *when cold air touches the larynx*. This remedy is very *sensitive to draughts*. Over-sensitivity characterises the remedy. It can be seen in the acute as *irritability*.

SUPPURATION – EPITHELIAL *and LYMPH GLANDS. INNER TUBE –> LYMPHATIC SYSTEM. Where it is inflammatory look out for the itch, described as scratchy.*

Ignatia is a contrary remedy so the *lump sensation* is only there when they are not swallowing, although sometimes they will try and try to swallow it but cannot. Like *Lachesis* they can *swallow solids better* than empty swallowing, but *Lachesis* is a remedy of congestive swelling whereas *Ignatia* is a remedy of spasm. There is often an emotional cause that lowers their vitality, e.g. grief bringing a lump to their throat! The tonsils may be swollen and ulcerated. There are *choking spasms* that are *relieved after taking a deep breath.* They will not eat simple foods. They will ask for illogical foods such as tomato ketchup, *sour foods.*

INFLAMMATION -> SPASM of involuntary muscle -> local swelling -> ulceration. *The emotional context resulting in spasm shows the involvement here of the autonomic nervous system.*

Lachesis may develop a sore throat from *continual use of the voice.* This is the remedy of the teacher or the singer. Catarrh produced to protect the connective tissue gives the sensation of *a lump that rises but is swallowed down again, only to rise again.* The patient tends to choke when *swallowing empty* but liquid is swallowed more easily and *solids swallowed with ease.* This remedy is prepared from the venom of the Surukuku snake! Snakes make an art of swallowing solids. The breath is foul showing suppuration at the very least, often sepsis. When they open the mouth wide *the pain extends to the ear.* Think of the snake's open jaws! *First the left then the right side is affected.*

Individualistically this patient is *sensitive to slight pressure but better from firm pressure* – that is why they can swallow solid food better. It makes firm contact with the sides of the throat.

This is a deeper disturbance than the remedies above. The system may become involved generally so the patient may appear dopey in the morning, *worse after sleep,* and get more irritable as the day goes on. They have a nasty temper and as they feel poisoned so they lash out with their tongue poisoning others with their *sarcasm.*

SUPPURATION – Local (PARTICULAR) -> system (GENERAL).

This is a remedy of congestion showing suppuration extending from the area to affect surrounding structures such as the ear but also affecting systemically.

Mercurius is a remedy that *salivates copiously* so they want *to swallow all the time.* As they do so there is a *stitching pain extending to the right ear.* Often the catarrh produces a sensation *as if a piece of apple were stuck in the throat.* There are large lumps of catarrh in the throat or quinsies with copious catarrh and *foul breath* with a *metallic taste.* When they *swallow liquid it comes back up through the nose.* These patients are always taking sore throats when *the weather changes* or perhaps *after a draught* as in *Hepar sulphuris.* They *sweat copiously with the pain.*

SUPPURATION – Local (INNER TUBE and LYMPH GLANDS) -> MINOR ORGAN involving SWEAT GLANDS (Skin as system) *This is severe suppuration. It is a syphilitic remedy capable of much degeneration and necrosis. There is a lack of integrity.*

Pulsatilla is a remedy of mumps where the *parotid glands swell.* Other glands swell causing tonsillitis. Pain and swelling may move from *right to left.* There is *difficulty swallowing* because the throat is *so dry. Food sticks in the throat* and cannot pass because the lining is not lubricated and yet they are *thirstless.* The dryness has a *stuffy, congested feeling* so they *dislike heat* and *want fresh air.* When they are up and about the catarrh moves so it is *worse in the morning.* The symptoms arise *after they get their feet wet* or, like *Mercurius,* at any change in the weather, particularly *from cold to warm weather.* They are *aggravated going into warm rooms* meaning they feel more stuffy and sore.

SUPPURATION – second level of defence. INNER TUBE -> LYMPHATIC SYSTEM. *Here we start with local congestion and dryness affecting epithelial tissue and glands. Stuffiness.*

Rhus toxicodendron is a remedy of inflammation and of strained ligaments and tendons, connective tissue. In some sore throats of *Rhus toxicodendron* the soft palate at the back of the throat is *swollen, red and itchy*. Tonsils may also be swollen with *yellow pus* so it is *difficult to swallow*. This may occur *after they get a soaking, e.g. falling in the river*, or *are severely chilled after overheating (ice cream after roasting on the beach)*. The voice may be affected so it is *hoarse*. The voice may also be affected through *overuse* as in *Lachesis*.

INFLAMMATION -> SUPPURATION – OUTER TUBE and INNER TUBE epithelial tissue -> MIDDLE TUBE connective tissue. Irritation as ITCH becomes General RESTLESSNESS.

Silicea is very similar to *Pulsatilla* in many ways but is deeper and *moves from left to right*. Vitality is lower so they may have recurrent sore throats *whenever the weather changes*. The *breath is foul in a sour way*, the tonsils suppurate and are so swollen that the *Silicea* patient *gags and retches. Food is ejected back up through the nose* when they try to swallow, as in *Mercurius*. They are *sensitive to draughts*, as in *Hepar sulphuris*. Also as in *Hepar sulphuris*, the mucus membrane dries to produce *stick-like sensations in the throat*. Unlike *Hepar sulphuris* and like *Pulsatilla* they are *mild and gentle, peevish and sorry for themselves* when ill.

SUPPURATION is localised into the EPITHELIAL lining tissue and the LYMPH GLANDS. However, Silicea can go deeper into the MAJOR ORGAN of the lungs or into the MIDDLE TUBE as rheumatism. Slow Healer because so little vitality.

EXERCISE

Make a table of comparison of the above remedies.

Here are some headings you could use:

> Modalities
> Types of pain
> Location
> Exciting Causes
> Strange, Rare and Peculiar symptoms

SOME INTERESTING INDIVIDUALITY IN SORE THROATS

I have limited the number of remedies to the most common and hence available at home or in the First Aid Box!

PHARYNX	
Pain alternates sides	*Lachesis, Lac canium*
As if an apple core stuck there	*Mercurius, Phytolacca*
Burning sensation swallowing	*Arsenicum, Hepar sulphuris*
Choking spasms > bending backwards	*Hepar sulphuris, Lachesis*
Spasms from drinking water	*Belladonna, Cantharis, Hyoscyamus, Stramonium*
Throat feels coated	*Pulsatilla*
Extending to the ear	*Hepar sulphuris, Lachesis, Mercurius, Phytolacca*
Food sticks in the throat	*Pulsatilla*
As if a hair in the throat	*Kali bichromium, Silicea*
Grasps the throat	*Aconite, Drosera, Phosphorus*
Hollow, empty sensation	*Lachesis, Phytolacca*
Itching	*Nux vomica, Rhus toxicodendron*
As if a lump	*Hepar sulphuris, Ignatia, Lachesis, Pulsatilla*
Lump rises and is swallowed again	*Lachesis*
As if a splinter (or fishbone)	*Argentum nitricum, Hepar sulphuris, Phytolacca, Silicea*
< talking	*Aconite, Bryonia, Ignatia, Mercurius,*
< sweets	*Lachesis*
> sweets	*Arsenicum*
	Phosphorus
< acids	*Antimonium crudem, Sepia*
Ulceration	*Arsenicum, Lachesis, Mercurius, Nux vomica*
Full of vesicles	*Cantharis*
As if a worm wriggling in throat	*Pulsatilla*
> lying on the back	*Lachesis*
Slimy	*Belladonna, Lachesis, Mercurius, Pulsatilla*
LARYNX	
< bending backwards	*Belladonna, Lachesis*
< blowing the nose	*Causticum*
Constricting spasm	*Aconite, Belladonna, Ignatia, Phosphorus*
on scratching auditory canal	*Silicea*
while talking	*Drosera*
< coughing	*Belladonna, Nux vomica, Phosphorus, Pulsatilla*
As if a crumb in	*Lachesis*
As if a feather in	*Drosera*
As if a foreign substance	*Belladonna*
Paralysis	*Causticum, Lachesis*
As if a plug	*Lachesis*
Rattling in the larynx	*Hepar sulphuris, Ipecacuanha*
As if there was a skin in	*Phosphorus*
Tickling	*Aconite, Ignatia, Lachesis, Nux vomica, Phosphorus, Pulsatilla, Silicea*

Remedies

Belladonna

This is a remedy of Fire. It produces Inflammation and fever. It is a remedy of really healthy people, especially children, because it represents this first level of defence. The activity of the blood is increased so we find the characteristic symptoms are:
- bright redness
- heat – *so intense it radiates from them*
- swelling
- throbbing pain
- *pains shooting upwards.*

The movement of blood is *up towards the head* so a keynote symptom is *visibly throbbing carotid artery* – look into the angle of the jaw. *Belladonna* is a *right sided* remedy. The fiery heat is seen in a *bright red face*. With so much heat there is also *dryness – no sweat*. The *Belladonna* fever is so hot you can *feel the heat without touching the skin*. The heat warms up the cool clothes applied to the brow! The temperature rises very high but you know all is well after giving the remedy, even if it goes higher immediately, because the patient starts to sweat within minutes. When the sweat starts the body cools down and the crisis is over.

The same symptoms may be found locally whether you have hit your thumb with a hammer, been stung by a bee or have appendicitis, earache or swollen tonsils. The local part swells, is bright red and throbs. If the thumb is affected the pains may shoot up the arm. Elsewhere, pains may appear as spasms. The part is *very sensitive to touch* and further *heat* of any kind. In the headache or fever, an individualistic symptom is *worse jar*. This includes anything that jolts them even mis-stepping – suddenly finding a step they did not know was there, or stepping off the pavement.

When disturbed on the Mental and Emotional level, they will turn on you with an irritability or even violent snarl. Children may *bite*. Adults also bite when you remember that this was the remedy Samuel Hahnemann used to pioneering work with *mania* in the asylums of 18th century Germany. Mania in fever is *delirium – they see monsters*. In temperament, this is a remedy of Rage – *hot-headedness.*

This remedy was considered specific for rabies and although we seldom see this today, it may help you remember some of the individualistic symptoms in severe fever. Children in high fevers may go into *convulsions, bending the spine backwards as in meningitis,* or *delirium* – the remedy may be used for the high dry fever of measles before the spots come out. Like the sweat, once the spots are out, most of the danger is over. In delirium, the *Belladonna* patient is *wild,* the eyes are *staring, the pupils dilated.* They *see monsters,* have a *terror of dogs* and *water* and may even froth at the mouth in rage. Unlike the *Aconite* patient, the terror is quickly covered by defensive rage, so they lash out at you, striking and biting.

It is not a pretty picture, even if very quickly relieved by *Belladonna*. Thankfully it is not common these days. The *Belladonna* fever is common but more likely to occur *after the head has been exposed to the sun* or is chilled by going outside *in the cold with wet hair,* or after a sudden soaking out in the rain without a hat. The head is most vulnerable to cold, wet conditions.

Since it is a remedy of *spasm in circular muscles (sphincters and ducts),* it is often seen in gall stone colic or when kidney stones are passed where the excruciating violent pain gives rise to a waterfall of sweat when *Belladonna* is given, and the stone is passed. *Belladonna* dilates ducts to let the stone pass just as it dilates the pupils in a fever (or the iris of the beautiful lady).

Belladonna is such an acute remedy that we seldom see it in deeper pathology. The Homoeopath sees three levels of disease – Sensation, Dysfunction and Pathology. These represent deepening stages of disturbance. *Belladonna* acts on the first level of Sensation characterised by pain and inflammation. Where it enters the Dysfunction level it is evident as spasm, particularly in circular muscles. Remedies that work at this level have more Individuality visible as keynotes and Strange, Rare and Peculiar symptoms. Often this is seen in their *Time modalities. Belladonna* is < 3pm.

Now, what in Anatomy and Physiology could possibly explain a time modality? The Acupuncturist has a body clock of times when major organs reach their peak re performance and their zenith when illness is most likely to strike. In more chronically diseased people, these days, *Belladonna* can often be seen to aggravate at 3am, which is very different from in Hahnemann's day. When it aggravates at 3am we do not see the fiery fever in the head but a lesser expression in a minor organ such as an ear. Come back and consider this when we have studied Vitality and Potency in Lesson 5.

SELF TEST

1. A keynote symptom we had said is a special symptom that belongs almost exclusively to one remedy, sometimes 2-3, so it helps us identify the remedy quickly. List 5 keynotes of *Belladonna*.

2. What are the four aggravating modalities mentioned above?

3. Sketch a picture of the raging *Belladonna* in fever. Now is your chance to show off your artistic skills!

4. Of what two things is a *Belladonna* patient terrified?

5. You have hit your thumb with a hammer. Describe what you saw and felt, how you reacted if you were a *Belladonna* patient.

Check the answers by reviewing the text.

Lachesis

Lachesis is a very different remedy from *Belladonna* although its action is also through the blood. It will be very useful to study it here to show the very different types of symptoms that arise.

The Surukuku snake is one of the viper type, found in South America. The venom causes blood to clot. Death usually arises when the blood reaching the heart is clotted. If we relate this to the constitution, the patient is often called a *venous* type because insufficient capacity to reabsorb fluid gives rise to congestion and slowness in circulation. The oedematous extremities ultimately affect the heart. *Lachesis* is one of the Homoeopath's major remedies of heart disease. It is a more chronic remedy than *Belladonna* so illness is slow to develop.

The *Lachesis* patient grows progressively more sluggish as the circulation slows down. In the end stages they will produce *bulbous blue varicose veins*, discoloured black legs from the ankles up, *varicose ulcers* with *black coagulated blood* but this may be many years ahead. The earlier picture is dullness of consciousness, < *after eating, inability to wake up in the morning,* migraines as the blood becomes more congested before a menstrual period. The period itself may be extremely painful *until flow is established.* Then the flow is likely to be clotted or even *thick, tarry black.* The pelvic cavity is bloated and congested, < *for the pressure of clothes.*

As we move more deeply into chronic disease, into the constitution, the modalities become greater indicators of Individuality than the Exciting Cause. Like the snake that goes to sleep after eating, the *Lachesis* patient is *very dopey after eating* or *worse heat.* It is worse for anything that further slows down the flow. We say that it is > *discharge* whether that is sweat, menstrual blood, bowel motions, etc. When they are very congested they are worse for anything that starts the flow but ultimately better for it so we need to be aware of the stage of congestion to read the symptom picture accurately. It is one of the remedies that *sleep into the aggravation* because sleep slows down metabolism and it is difficult for them to get going again, so they are much *worse in the morning after sleep.* It is a remedy of liver sluggishness – the liver stores and transforms energy, glucose to glycogen and vice versa – so they are worse for anything that slows down the liver – *< eating, < alcohol, < menstruation.* It may be a useful remedy for alcoholism when the liver is under attack and circulation is sluggish. The viciousness and selfishness that dominates craving may construe a stereotype similar to that of the *Lachesis* patient's temperament.

Liver sluggishness produces *awful constipation* and severe headaches that typically *move from left to right.* As in all congestion the pain is *throbbing.* Often there is nausea, always the pain is < heat and the patient is dull in consciousness. Usually the headache occurs before the menstrual period when the liver has extra work to do in expelling oestrogen from the system.

Snakes have always been associated with women's fertility in mythology. The *Lachesis* symptoms would vindicate this relation. Menstruation is discharge and as long as it occurs all is well, > discharge, but the blood is clotted. When the skin of the uterus is sloughed off it is not dissolved to pass painlessly out. The clots may be so big or the process so inadequate that great chunks of Endometrium attempt to pass. As the cervix is not sufficiently open the uterus goes into spasm. So the greatest pain is before the flow commences giving rise to the symptom *better at commencement of flow*. More than that, in severe cases the pain is described as *labour-like,* or *as if the contents of the abdomen would be expelled.* Many *Lachesis* patients find childbirth a dawdle! In such a severe situation, there are other symptoms of congestion – fluid retention gives rise to swollen breasts especially on the left side, distended abdomen, oedema in ankles and fingers. Liver congestion leads to constipation relieved after the flow starts and headaches with nausea. During this premenstrual state when the abdomen is affected we may see other keynote modalities that reflect the nature of the snake. They cannot bear any tight clothing of any form. The symptom is << *slightest touch and > for firm pressure.* The snake hears through vibrations and is rendered harmless if grasped around the neck. You will not catch this patient wearing a polo neck sweater.

In the sore throat it is this modality that leads to the Individuality of *< empty swallowing > swallowing solids* that can be felt to firmly press against the sides of the throat. It is this sensitivity that leads to the strange *sensation of lumps or balls.* Usually these are felt to rise. When the snake eats its meal is one large lump that gets progressively smaller as it passes along the digestive tract. In indigestion the heart feels like a lump in the centre of the chest. The catarrh of the sore throat is a *ball that rises up* to be swallowed down only to rise again. The lump in the abdomen may be an impacted bowel or a false pregnancy. This is a major remedy of fibroids that are massive lumps felt in the uterus at physical examination. Even the varicose veins are bulbous lumps. And note how these started as sensations, became involved in dysfunction in digestion them became actual and real in uterine pathology. The lumps or balls are part of the Individuality of *Lachesis.*

When we come to menopause, *Lachesis* may be important remedy to consider because here is its Essence (the tone of the Individuality that runs through all symptoms) – flow ceases. There are symptoms of distension, water retention, headaches, *flushes upward, night sweats about the head and chest, palpitations.* We have seen how the clotting of the blood will eventually affect the heart in snakebite. Here we see the link between the heart and the uterus. To the Acupuncturist the heart is the extraordinary vessel. It is a solid organ and its counterpart is the hollow uterus. In studying the unfoldment of chronic disease I find this explains a pattern that arises often in menopause. Some types of patient have palpitations, other do not. When we also have left sidedness in the headaches, it pays to investigates *Lachesis* more closely. There is often high blood pressure relieved by nosebleeds. Flushes of heat move up to the head and migraines are more common. As a major heart remedy *Lachesis* symptom of Individuality is a fear to move *in case the heart should stop beating.* It is slow to affect the heart building up through congestion of the extremities in varicose veins and oedemas. They will become sluggish after eating and eventually have breathing difficulties on exercise because fluid builds up in the lungs. It is not a nice end.

Homoeopathically we do not have to wait that long because the remedy is indicated in the temperament well before it gets to the pathological level. Like the snake the personality is *shy and retiring* but increasingly becoming *suspicious* of others' goodwill towards them. One patient even described herself as a snake in the grass in how she went about getting her own back on the local minister. This is a very deep remedy where the inferiority complex often arises from an unpleasant childhood. They may be so badly damaged that they become *malicious* and vindictive, seeking revenge, and *poisoning the air with their brooding presence.* Their *sarcasm* is biting, although *loquacity* may enable them to get it out, or nag. They may be dour and oppressed expecting the worst. They may find salvation in religion but it may be of the Calvinistic type where much authority keeps their instincts under control, where law rules. Like Calvin they have a sense of predestination, *a foreboding of doom.* When very deeply disturbed, as in *grief* or *disappointed love,* they may see the loved one beside them and even talk to him/her as if alive. From the subconscious *they hear voices telling them what to do* – this might give you a different angle on Psycho! It is one of our remedies of deep depression – before menses, after pregnancy, after grief or disappointed love, at menopause, after a repressed childhood. It is the kind of depression in which the self is attacked through low self esteem.

As you can see some remedies go very deep indeed. We call these **constitutional remedies** because they deal with the fundamental causes of chronic disease. More of that later.

ACTIVITY

If you do not know much about snakes, you will understand this remedy better if you study them a little? Visit a zoo, read a book. Good luck!

> **EXERCISE**
>
> 1. Put the italic type symptoms into columns headed Strange, Rare and Peculiar, Mental and Emotional, General, Particular. Note, Keynotes can be found in any group.
>
> 2. List **six** aggravating modalities and **two** ameliorating modalities.

Lachesis

STRANGE, RARE AND PECULIAR	MENTAL AND EMOTIONAL	GENERAL	PARTICULAR

Belladonna

STRANGE, RARE AND PECULIAR	MENTAL AND EMOTIONAL	GENERAL	PARTICULAR

Lesson 4

SELF TEST

1. Which is not true of the pains of *Belladonna*?
   - Shooting ☐
   - Throbbing ☐
   - Stabbing ☐
   - Burning ☐

2. What does not accompany the fever of *Belladonna*?
   - Sweat ☐
   - Dryness ☐
   - Redness ☐
   - Violent pain ☐

3. What does not accompany the menopause of the *Lachesis* patient?
   - Hot flushes upward ☐
   - Clotted black blood ☐
   - Palpitations ☐
   - Food allergies ☐

4. What is the most common type of heart disease in the *Lachesis* patient?
   - Angina ☐
   - Congestive heart disease ☐
   - Heart murmur ☐
   - Arrhythmia ☐

5. What are the symptoms of the *Belladonna* rabies?
   - Sweat ☐
   - Fear of water ☐
   - Foaming at the mouth ☐
   - Biting ☐

6. Which of the following is a keynote of *Lachesis*?
   - < after eating ☐
   - labour-like pain as if contents expelled ☐
   - sensation of lumps ☐
   - << slightest touch, > firm pressure ☐
   - suspicious ☐

7. What may cause the *Belladonna* fever?
   - Getting the head chilled ☐
   - Getting the feet wet ☐
   - Too much sun ☐
   - A cold wind ☐

8. Which adjectives describe the *Belladonna* patient?
   - Fearful ☐
   - Enraged ☐
   - Touchy ☐
   - Wild ☐

9. Which adjectives describe the *Lachesis* patient?
   - Suspicious ☐
   - Loquacious ☐
   - Vindictive ☐
   - Shy ☐
   - Gloomy ☐

10. *Lachesis* affects the venous system. Which symptoms indicate this?
    - Bulbous, blue veins ☐
    - Constipation ☐
    - Dopey after eating ☐
    - < in the morning ☐

Check the answers by reviewing the text.

THROAT PAIN REPERTORY

Right sided	*acon, arn,* **ars, bell, bry, coloc,** *hep, ogn, merc,* **nux v, puls,** *sil*
Extending to left	acon, bell
Left sided	acon, *arn, bry, coloc, cimic,* gels, hep, ign, **lach,** *merc,* **sep,** *sil*
Extending to right	acon, **lach,** *rhus t*
Extending to the ear	*bell,* bry, *hep,* ign, *lach,* merc, nat m,
On swallowing	*gels,* lach, merc, **nux v**
Pain burning	**acon,** *arn,* **ars,** *bell,* **canth,** coloc, *gels, hep,* lach, merc, **nat m,** nux v, puls, *rhus t, sep,* sil
rawness	acon, ars, **bell,** *coloc, hep,* ign, *lach,* merc, nat m, **nux v,** *puls, sep,* sil
sore	acon, *ars,* **bell,** *gels,* **ign,** lach, *led,* **merc,** nat m, *nux v,* puls, *rhus t, sep,* sil
as from a splinter	**hep,** ign, *lach,* merc, *nat m,* sil
stitching	**acon,** arn, ars, **bell,** *bry,* **hep,** *ign,* lach, led, merc, nat m, nux v, **puls,** rhus t, sep, sil
< cold air	bell, *hep, merc,* nux v
< on coughing	acon, hep, *lach,* nat m, *nux v, sep, sil*
< on speaking	acon, bell, merc, rhus t
< swallowing	acon, **ars, bell,** *bry,* gels, **hep,** ign, *lach,* led, **merc,** nat m, *nux v,* puls, *rhus t,* sep, *sil*
< empty swallowing	ars, *bell,* bry, hep, **lach,** *merc,* nux v, *puls, rhus t,* ruta, sep
< warm drinks	**lach**
> warm drinks	**ars, hep,** nux v, *rhus t*
LARYNX	
In morning on waking	*nux v* sep
< bending head backwards	*bell,* bry, **lach,** *sil*
on coughing	bell, **bry,** ign, nat m, *nux v,* puls
Pain burning	*ars,* gels, lach, merc, *puls,* sep
rawness	*acon,* arn, *nat m,* ruta, sep, sil
stitching	acon, bell, hep, led,
< on coughing	*ars, bell,* bry, **nux v, puls,** sep
< inspiration	**acon, hep,** sil
from talking	*ars, nat m*
as if a plug in the larynx	bell, *hep, lach,* sep
Tickling in larynx	**acon,** *arn,* ars, bell, *bry,* cimic, coloc, hep, ign, **lach,** led, *merc,* **nat m, nux v,** *puls, rhus t,* **sep,** *sil*
Hoarse voice from talking	arn, lach, *nat m,* **rhus t**

READING

George Vithoulkas   Homoeopathy and the New Man   Thorsons
A general introduction to Homoeopathy in modern language.

Harris Coulter   Modern Medicine and Homoeopathic Science
I usually recommend this introductory book to the more 'scientific' minded.

THOUGHT TO PONDER

The material organism, without the vital force, is capable of no sensation, no function, no self-preservation; it derives all sensations and performs all the functions of life solely by means of the immaterial being (the vital force or principle) which animates the material organism in health and in disease.

Para 10, The Organon of the Rational Art of Healing
Samuel Hahnemann

LESSON 5   Earache

Aims: To look at what happens when disease moves into the minor organ.
To study more about the acute ailment.
To study more about levels of defence as related to vitality and potency.
To study the three factors of disease – predisposition, exciting cause and constitution.
To relate acute and chronic disease.
To identify the Aggravation.
To study the homoeopathic remedies *Silicea, Hepar sulphuris* and *Mercurius*.
To study Hering's four Laws of Cure.
To begin a study of levels of the disease process – sensation, dysfunction and structural change.

Keywords used:

predisposition	suppuration
constitution	miasms
inflammatory response	minor organ
exciting cause	dysfunction and structural level of disease
vitality	aggravation

In this lesson we are moving on to another category of acute disease. In dealing with headaches we looked at exciting and maintaining causes and how head pain might be related to the underlying structure or constitutional disease. In looking at sore throats we introduced the idea of level of defence as in inflammation or suppuration. We will continue these themes here but we will also move on to look at the acute in a minor organ in terms of the constitution.

The Structure of the Ear

The ear is a sense organ specialised to enable communication with the outside world. It is divided into three parts: the outer ear, the middle ear and the inner ear.

The outer ear is that kidney shape we draw on faces! It is fleshy supported by cartilage acting as a collector of sound like a satellite disc. Sound is channelled down a passage to the eardrum, or tympanic membrane, where it vibrates. I like to give it its name because it reminds me of the sensitivity of the skin of the timpani drums in the orchestra.

On the other side of the tympanic membrane is the middle ear. Three little bones connect the tympanic membrane to the inner ear. These are named from their shapes, the hammer, anvil and stirrup (in Latin of course). Also in the middle ear is an open passage to the throat called the Eustachian tube. This allows air pressure to equalise on either side of the tympanic membrane. You will have knowledge of this process from a lift or aeroplane when changing height rapidly – the ears pop. Loss of hearing occurs when the tympanic membrane is pierced so it cannot vibrate or when catarrh clogs the middle ear preventing the vibration. More serious deafness may occur with age when the bones become arthritic and fail to carry the vibration,

The inner ear is where the sound is received and transferred to the nervous system via an organ called the cochlea that looks like a snail shell. Lining this curled-up tube are hairs which are vibrated by the passing sound waves so causing nerve impulses in the auditory nerve. When it is damaged we might not hear high frequencies of sound or may hear these all the time as in tinnitus. Surrounding the cochlea are three loops called the semicircular canals that are filled with fluid. These are so arranged that the position of the fluid informs us whether we are upside down, leaning to the left or right, etc like the horizon of an aeroplane. Problems here lead to dizziness and lack of orientation.

What is Earache?

A simple earache may occur in a relatively healthy individual who is exposed to a fierce wind on a day at the seaside a little too early in the year. Beyond the very thin membrane of the eardrum is the inside of the body. Indeed at this point we are inside the skull. After such exposure almost anyone could produce a defensive inflammatory response. Inflammation is the first stage of disturbance when the redness and heat show excessive blood has been rushed to the area bringing heat primarily in this situation. In this case, we need help Nature only a little with a hot water bottle or a little heated almond oil in the ear – take care this is not too hot by first putting a little on the back of your hand. Covering the ears in cold weather may prevent the whole situation. The homeopathic remedies indicated are those of inflammation, and of conditions that come on very quickly and may resolve just as quickly, e.g. *Aconite, Belladonna*.

In the less healthy there is a deeper response producing catarrh. In some there is a tendency to produce excess secretion in the middle ear as a weak Location, or affinity in the first instance, whatever the exciting cause, e.g. *Pulsatilla, Silica*. In yet other remedies the catarrh creeps up extending from the upper respiratory system so it is a sign of deepening situation rather than weak Location, e.g. *Bryonia, Lachesis, Mercurius,* and also *Pulsatilla* at another level of expression. We need to study the progression of the disease. The type of pain may help as in the first (inflammatory) it is much more severe than on the second (suppurative). The first situation has more heat and a strong reaction to cold; the second may be described as a fullness that affects hearing.

Acute Illness and the Level of the Disease Process

Sometimes you notice that this child is prone to such disturbances as earache and perhaps the weather was not that cold – the Vital Force was *susceptible*. It may be in such cases that it is always the left ear although both may be equally exposed. Now, we have *Individuality* and are speaking of a weakness, or predisposition, to an exciting cause. The fact that the Vital Force has chosen a specific location, the *left* ear, indicates its action to express disturbance through specific channels, characteristic to this Vital Force. Left sided and < cold wind become part of the symptom picture. This is an *acute* in the homoeopathic sense. The Vital Force is disturbed and the Vital Force produces an acute illness.

Samuel Hahnemann describes an acute illness as something from which you either completely recover or die! Acute illness has a special place in Homoeopathy. It tells us more about the nature of the Vital Force and it tells us about the vitality of the Vital Force. A relatively healthy Vital Force, we have learned, produces illness on the first level of defence, inflammation. Good examples of this are the symptom pictures of *Aconite* and *Belladonna* in earache. The pains are throbbing and intense as blood attempts to restore heat. Usually the exciting cause comes from without as in exposure to cold weather. *Hepar sulphuris* and *Causticum* may also be indicated when the exciting cause is < cold weather but there action is 'deeper'.

On a deeper level, the acute occurs in the middle ear. This is slower to develop and will not be cured simply with a hot water bottle. The Vital Force is weaker and allows the disturbance to go deeper, into more complicated physiological structures or more serious defence actions. Catarrh arises as part of the second level of defence, suppuration. If you look carefully at this case it is not simple exposure. The vitality is lowered. The factors which lowered the vitality may be various, including Mental and Emotional symptoms such as shock. They bring us into a strange place of the relationship between psyche and soma. The effect of an Exciting Cause shows clearly the way in which the Vital Force operates. The Homoeopath says disease does not just appear. It needs the Predisposition from the constitutional weakness that tells us where the symptoms will manifest. It needs the exciting cause, that to which the Vital Force is susceptible, and we need lowered vitality. Exciting causes lower vitality because they strike at the Vital Force. However, vitality may be lowered previously or as part of the ongoing constitutional weakness needing the prod of the exciting cause to push the Vital Force just that little bit further to produce an acute.

It is also the case that the healthy Vital Force may produce the acute when energy rises and it has the energy to do so. This is a very unusual concept for those new to Homoeopathy. When crippled by chronic disease, miasms, the Vital Force is kept in a state of lowered health. It does not have the energy to correct the warp further so accommodates the disturbance by drawing it to a deeper level, hence the earache in the middle ear in this example. In its compromised state the Vital Force will leap at an opportunity to open the door and express the disease. However, rather than disable the whole on a general level, or in the physiological systems where vital functions may be compromised, the Vital Force may throw the disturbance out at the level of the *minor organ.* The exciting cause is thus a great friend! The Homoeopath welcomes such acutes as the level of the chronic disease changes immediately after the acute. Indeed the chronic symptom picture often appears after the acute when previously it was in latency. When this happens it may appear that the patient is worse. J. T. Kent emphasised that it is the symptoms that get worse and not the patient. How do we judge if this is so? As the healing process proceeds, the level on which the symptoms manifest should change according to Hering's Laws of Cure.

Many earaches do not fall into either of the acute categories mentioned but may accompany other illnesses such as colds. The ear may be involved only as the situation deepens and catarrh pushes into further structure, e.g. the sore throat of *Mercurius* and *Lachesis* often extend to the ear as the patient tries to swallow. This may be due to dryness or the encroaching up the Eustachian tube of the catarrh itself. In Homoeopathy this tells us the characteristic *modus operandi* as well as *location* or affinity of the indicated remedy.

The Aggravation

This seems a significant point to mention the homoeopathic aggravation. You will hear tell that it is good news when the symptoms get worse after treatment. I want you to hear me loud and clear that this is not so.

J. T. Kent distinguishes between the symptoms getting worse and the patient getting worse. As we will see below, vital processes should never be worsened after homoeopathic treatment. A vital process such as bleeding should not be aggravated. The aggravation of symptom is always according to Hering's four Laws of Cure. More specifically, what is aggravated illustrates the movement outwards of the symptoms. Within the constitutional symptom picture there are clear drains and channels along which the symptoms can expect to flow when vitality is increased. Usually these are indicated by previous illnesses. The aggravation is not arbitrary but entirely predictable from careful case taking – as long as the patient does not miss out anything significant in discussing previous health problems. There are occasions when the energy created by the homeopathic remedy is more than is needed to remove the visible symptoms. It will then dig deeper to affect old symptoms and conditions. On occasions when the energy moves too fast to expel disturbance it may sweep along creating new channels, like a stream, but along the lines of action of the remedy and at higher level of function or defence than previously.

When we give a homoeopathic remedy, our aim is not to 'cure' the patient but to stimulate the Vital Force into action to create a higher level of health than previously. In today's world that might mean simply raising the level at which the disease is manifest (i.e. more bronchitis to tonsillitis). More ideally that is just a step on the way. However, the Homoeopath works with the Vital Force so seldom gives more than one pill at a time and always watching the pattern of movement of symptoms to tell him/her what the Vital Force is doing and what treatment is then necessary, if any. Thus it is important for the patient to carefully note any change in symptoms after a remedy and to report back on their progress for further assessment.

Vitality

Vitality is one of the three factors needed for symptoms to manifest, i.e. predisposition, exciting cause and lowered vitality. Also, an assessment of vitality determines the potency used since the more energy the patient has then the faster the symptoms will move in the direction of cure, or the greater the amount and the swifter toxins, the products of catabolism, will move through the drains and channels to the exterior – in other words the more severe the aggravation. Thus the Homoeopath needs to consider measurement of vitality.

We usually say that the faster the symptoms appear after exposure then the greater the vitality. Here, we have studied how inflammatory symptoms, which are usually more severe and serious, indicate higher vitality than slower moving suppurative symptoms. We have looked at severity of symptoms as expressed in how deeply the disturbance has penetrated from the outer tube of the skin inwards to the respiratory, digestive and urinary tracts, noting the difference between tissue and system. At the system level dysfunction is a more serious process than local manifestations. The most serious situation occurs when symptoms are expressed in the vital organs. Of course each situation is unique and such rules are only a guide. The Homoeopath will always consider the Total Symptom Picture.

Then, to complicate matters further, some remedies are slower than others. A 6th or 30th potency of one remedy may represent an entirely different level of energy than in another. It is a lifetime's study. Hence, in these lessons, I have added potency to symptoms to give you some idea.

Remedies for Earache

Aconite   after exposure to cold conditions there is *tearing pain* in the *left* ear. The child will be very *distressed and restless* because of the intensity of the pain. The young child may even show the fear of *Aconite*. The part may be red and hot. It will be *better for the application of heat*.

A single dose of the 30th potency will disperse the pain rapidly. Sleep will ensue. The 30th potency is used because of the speed of onset, lack of complication and violence of the symptom picture. Only a single dose should be necessary if the correct remedy is selected.

Belladonna   The patient will describe the pain here as *shooting or throbbing*. They will be so irritable they will *easily fly into a rage*. Once again the ear may look red and feel *hot after exposure to cold* but this time it will be the *right* ear that is affected.

Once again the 30th potency will restore calm rapidly. As above, the 30th potency is used because of the speed of onset, lack of complication and violence of the symptom picture. Only a single dose should be necessary if the correct remedy is selected.

Pulsatilla   This remedy may start on *exposure to cold, wet weather*. Catarrh is produced, building up pressure in the inner ear so *throbbing pains* result. It is the *right* ear that is affected but sometimes the disturbance moves to the left ear. The adult will *moan for sympathy*, the child will be *clingy and demanding*. Since they become like wet rags this remedy is often easy to spot. If the acute remains at the inflammatory level after exposure, an S R & P symptom may occur, *as if a wind blew through the ear*. At the suppurative stage the modality is *worse coming into a warm room*.

Now we have 2 levels indicated showing that this remedy can go deeper – that the symptom picture may present in different forms. We need skill to analyse the case to work out what is happening to the Vital Force and, in particular, how much energy it has for cure.

One dose of the 30th potency will cure after exposure to cold, wet conditions when the pain is right sided, i.e. clear exciting cause plus individuality and no complications such as other symptoms outside the ear.

One dose of the 200th potency may be indicated by the S R & P symptom *as if a wind were blowing through the ear*. It may also be required if the 30th potency has had no effect after 1-2 hours.

Where the pain has moved to the left side, the 200th potency may be needed if there are no other complications. Otherwise this or the strong presence of a modality may represent a slower Vital Force that is more deeply disturbed and therefore requires a repeat dose of the 6th potency (2-3X) to raise the energy level to the 30th potency. Giving the higher potency in this instance would create severe aggravation, which you do not want in the ear where catarrh may be present – with the energy of a 200th potency behind it, it may exit by the shortest route, i.e. through the eardrum! Return to the 30th potency will be indicated by simpler if more inflammatory symptoms, e.g. more heat and less catarrh. Repetition of the dose needs a Homoeopath who can skilfully read and analyse the symptom picture.

Silica is very similar to *Pulsatilla* in its symptom picture. The acute arises from *exposure to cold damp*. Once again they will be *moany* or *clingy* but this time it is the *left* side that is first affected. This is a deeper remedy. They are well aware of their tendency to catch colds so they are often spotted *wearing a hat!* The *Silica* patient is *stubborn* too.

The 30th potency is indicated by the 3 symptoms above, Exciting Cause, Location and Mental and Emotional symptoms, but this is a slow remedy so give it time to work: 4-6 hours. Do not speed up the Vital Force or interfere without clear indicating symptoms. Not only is this another catarrhal remedy, it is one of rapid centrifugal action! For this reason leave the 200th potency to the experienced Homoeopath who can accurately interpret the vitality of the Vital Force.

Lachesis Ear problems often start as a result of throat problems usually in *Autumn* or when the body has to adapt to *change to colder weather*. The swollen glands of this remedy start on the *left* side although they may migrate *to the right. Swallowing increases the pain.*

Heat makes them irritable. If the ear problem is allowed to deepen there may be *singing noises that are better when he/she puts a finger in the ear.* If it deepens yet further there will be a *smelly, bloody discharge* – the eardrum has burst at this point.

This is a remedy that may develop *abscesses in the mastoid area* so treatment early on is essential.

Leave this patient to the expert Homoeopath who may select one dose of the 30th potency where there is an exciting cause and throbbing pain still on the left side (primary location) indicating inflammation. Repeat doses of the 6th potency may be used because this is a destructive syphilitic miasm picture as indicated by the smell and bloody discharge. Where swallowing increases the pain, it often indicates the presence of catarrh, i.e. the second stage of suppuration.

When the singing noises or tinnitus are present there is nerve involvement (the inner ear) that needs urgent attention, as does pain in the mastoid process.

Mercurius Brought on by *change in the weather*, there is a stabbing pain in the *right* ear. There is an *urge to swallow* at first as catarrh builds up but this remedy progresses on to a *smelly discharge* that is *often bloody*. The smell is *foul*, of decay. There may be a *sensation as if cold water is running out of the ear.*

This is a remedy of lowered vitality but its essential pattern is collapse of integrity – it is another remedy of the syphilitic miasm. See how deeply the disturbance is expressed. The 30th potency is used to give a clear shape to the pattern, i.e. to contain it, but that is fine in the first stage only before it proceeds to the foul discharge stage. As the catarrh builds up, the aggravation will be worse, and will be even worse in the necrotic stage. There may be a better Individuality for *Mercurius corrosive* at this point as it has a stronger symptom picture of necrosis.

Hepar Sulphuris *Exposure to cold dry winds* produces first inflammation. This is *dry and raw* in the throat *as if a stick* is there. *Much yellow catarrh* is produced. Eventually when the eardrum bursts there is much yellow offensive pus *smelling of old cheese*. There is great *sensitivity to touch* and *movement* of the part, i.e. swallowing. This is a *very irritable* patient who will have covered the ear with a scarf *to keep out draughts*.

One dose of the 30th potency will cure if you can catch it at the first stage where there is dryness, rawness and the S R & P *as if a stick*. When the catarrh starts you may have to repeat the 6th potency to avoid externalising through the eardrum then finish with the 30th potency as the symptoms return to the first stage.

Where an eardrum has perforated, it may need repeat doses of the 30th potency to clear the catarrh then a 200th potency to heal the structural breach rapidly and to deepen the response into the preventive, i.e. to raise the underlying vitality so there are less weaknesses to relapse.

Kali muriaticum is one of the *stuffy* catarrh remedies, like *Pulsatilla* and *Silica*. They feel *pressure inside the ear* and *a crackling sound* coming from the catarrh. The *catarrh is bland and white*.

I would use the 30th potency because the Kali salts are very reactive. Once again we need to watch the change in the symptom picture. Here, because the inflammatory level is less visible (or less of a bother) you will see only the lingering of the catarrh, or a relapse, to indicate further treatment needed. The relapse is easier – give a single 200th potency for a bit more energy to the Vital Force. When the catarrh lingers you have more of a problem. To use the 200th now will surely aggravate whilst a repeat of the 30th will prolong cure and may awaken a few chronic symptoms. The answer here is to plus. Put the pill in a few millilitres of water and shake it jarringly to succuss the mixture then administer a little, keeping some to further succuss when you repeat the dose again. The time scale may be 4-6 hours between repetitions.

> **EXERCISE**
>
> Why do we always prescribe the 6th potency for a headache?
>
> Here are some clues: *Bilious = liver congestion*
>
> *Congestive = slow moving*
>
> *Tension = a build up but may need a simple break to relax.*
>
> (If deeper psychology then constitutional and needs more careful treatment.)
>
> There are some very effective homoeopathic remedies for pain relief but Homoeopathy is for cure not control of symptoms. We treat the TSP always!
>
> The exception to the rule? We might use *Gelsemium 30* in a *Natrum muriaticum* constitution simply to relieve the congestion of cerebrospinal fluid. We might use *Ignatia 30* or *Staphisagria 30* when a tension headache has a deeper emotional cause, grief, shock or indignation.

Remedies

Silicea

This is one of our oldest homoeopathic remedies, created by Samuel Hahnemann from river clay. It is also the quartz crystal found in sand and in volcanic rocks and used in glass. In nature we find it most commonly in the hard pericardium that protects the seed or in the tall grasses. In humans it is found in the hair and nails and in the lens of the eye. Now, what does that tell you of its properties? As hard as granite and as soft as clay. It occurs in crystalline and amorphous form. As the silicon chip it allows data to be imprinted and available to work with in a computer age.

Traditionally in Homoeopathy, this is seen as the remedy without backbone, *mild* and *yielding*. They are *chilly, phlegmatic types* who were seen in the TB age as spindly, sick weaklings prone to chest problems and rickets. As a constitutional type we see it in dwarfish sickly babies with an intolerance to milk, slow to close fontanelles and teething problems. They may be anxious with small angular heads, *startling at the least noise*, looking around to get their bearings. Often the abdomen is swollen with wind. Even as adults, thin and weedy looking, they may still have a large swollen abdomen showing poor digestion.

As toddlers and young children they are the *shy* watchers who stay on the edge of things but they are extremely perceptive and most often very intelligent although we do use this remedy for slowness to develop mental faculties (what was once called imbecility). They are extremely *sensitive* so stay on the edge of things *fearful* to join in. When they do join in they have sussed out how to do it. They may be held back from trying many new pursuits because of *fear of failure*. *Lack of grit* is a term most often used to describe their essence. They run out of energy easily so are more likely to know they might not be able to complete something and hold back because they do not want to be noticed.

One patient fell from her wheel chair and thereafter confined herself to it fearful to try again. Another child watched classmates play on the roof for some time before she had worked out it was safe to join them. This brings out one of their most characteristic symptoms, *stubbornness*. It will be done in their time, if at all.

They are deep thinkers. The cheery child will happily engage you on philosophical questions such as what happens when we die. Although shy they will take everything in and describe it to you afterwards in precise detail. I am reminded of the woman in Aldous Huxley's novel "Chrome Yellow" who sat on the edge of the drawing room making detailed sketches of the participants in the social circus.

What kind of illnesses do they suffer from? It is a remedy of the nerves and nervous debilities. Often this combines with the weakness to produce ME in over-stressed types or after flu. In more acute ailments the nervous weakness we find some strange sensations, e.g. *a sensation of a hair on the tongue, sensitivity to draft especially about the head so they wear a hat*. It has *over-sensitivity of the sense organs in general but especially to noise*. This brings in an affinity for the ear!

The phlegmatic, weakly type means a great *sensitivity to cold and damp*. They *easily take colds*. They have recurrent colds, perhaps one after another. *Copious catarrh* may be white or yellow, or often green. There may be so much catarrh that *liquids come back up through the nose*. More usually the nose is blocked, the sinus are blocked. Swollen glands are on the left side but may extend to the right. *Left –> Right*. The ear is often involved making *a popping noise on swallowing*. There is so much catarrh there but, as in *Pulsatilla*, it is bland. This does not stop it suffocating so there is deafness or lack of taste.

I was called out to see one little chap with earache. The mother could tell me little and I was a bit flummoxed until I realised there he was in his pyjamas with a balaclava helmet on his head. The ear was left sided and recurrent on exposure to the slightest cold damp. This is an important remedy to remember in ear problems where there is perforation or even involvement of the mastoid process as in mastoiditis.

Silica is a very slow acting remedy so is useful for weak slow constitutions that may produce long ongoing troubles. In First Aid we used it for wounds *stubborn to heal*. There is not enough energy to heal.

The relaxation (weakness) of tissue affecting the lymphatic system is found in constitutional symptoms such as *night sweats*, especially about the forehead. The foot sweat may be so *offensive, smelling of old cheese,* that it *rots the socks*. This is one of the main remedies of *suppressed foot sweat* where the result is *thick yellow discharges,* usually from the upper respiratory tract. On the subject of feet, the nails may be *distorted*, thickened, yellow and often crumbly. You could say there is no energy to take form. This may explain why there is so much catarrh and activity in the lymphatic system in the *Silicea* patient – it is the great sea of the body, the formless mass out of which in evolutionary terms the individualistic heart and circulation arises. Phlegmatic types are not renowned for egotism.

The lack of ability to take action is seen in such keynote symptoms as *bashful stool* where the stool starts to come out then retreats. There is a *yielding, mild nature, bashfulness* in general – the dwarf Bashful is a good stereotype of the *Silicea* patient. The lack of backbone is seen in such constitutional symptoms as *curvature of the spine.*

How can we explain why they have weak ankles and are good at maths? This is a polycrest which is a homoeopathic remedy with a very wide field of action so there are countless more symptoms and every homoeopathic remedy has two actions so in a well-proven remedy like *Silicea* you may see its opposite! What more do YOU need to know to use this remedy?

The exciting cause that would trigger an acute is cold and damp, or something that decreases the energy yet further. The odd energy patterns of timidity, advance and retreat, of vagueness to take form (in an acute this is to come to a crisis and resolve the situation) are the hallmarks (or essence) of the *Silicea* symptom picture.

Hepar sulphuris

This is one of the 'crotchety old colonel' remedies of extreme *irritability*. It is not calm or peaceful but driven. This is seen most clearly in the acute phase where it is characterised by *itch*.

Wounds are itchy as well as red and swollen. In this it resembles *Rhus toxicodendron*. In the *Hepar sulphuris* patient the wound quickly suppurates producing *yellow pus* with the characteristic *sour* smell *of old cheese*. Also, there is a *sensitivity to touch*, even of *cold air* that might pass over the wound. *Rhus toxicodendron* suppurates more slowly with greenish pus.

Coughs are another common acute when vitality drops. The *Hepar sulphuris* patient is sensitive to *cold, dry conditions*. The cold produced may be characterised by thick yellow catarrh with a 'scratchy' throat. As the *rawness* in the throat increases, there is a sensitivity of the parts touching – producing a sensation as if *a stick were stuck in the throat*. Or the *sensitivity to cold air causes the spasm of a cough*. The earache will occur where there is sudden exposure to cold dry conditions. It may start as inflammation then itch and will only produce discharge where the vitality is lower – then you will see the symptoms above, irritability and great sensitivity to touch even of a draught of air. In a more general illness such as flu even putting a hand outside of the bedclothes can cause the cough. *Hepar sulphuris* often occurs as an acute when *Silicea* and *Lycopodium* patients become run down. This is when we see another keynote symptom – they are extraordinarily *chilly*. It is the core heat, or vital heat, that is depleted so they may speak of taking a bath to warm up if *Silicea* or *Lycopodium* is the constitutional remedy. The constitutional *Hepar sulphuris* type is less likely to take a bath if only because any part raised from the bath water will feel very chilly.

In the constitutional type, the skin is very sensitive; it tends to dry. In eczema it can become raw and sore, easily excoriating so it becomes 'infected' and the yellow pus appears. More commonly, *Hepar sulphuris* is a remedy of herpetic eruptions – of cold sores, of chicken-pox and shingles. In all of these its Individuality is sour smelling yellow pus and very sensitive to touch, even of clothing.

Such sensitivity of the nerves and irritability produces a volatile type with a wicked temper akin to *Nux vomica* in that they will want to kill anyone who irritates them. They will be *impulsive* and *fickle*, so unpredictable. Since everything and everyone irritates them, you will find them *restless* and *quarrelsome*. Nothing pleases them. They are driven by the internal irritability to keep constantly on the move, in a *hurried manner*. One minute you might incline to *Nux vomica*, in another to *Rhus toxicodendron*, such is the similarity. Then you must remember the Individuality and the keynotes – *so chilly, sensitive to cold draughts, hurried*.

In a constitutional case the appetite may help – they *crave acids like vinegar* but acids may bring on the sore throats.

When they are more generally afflicted, as in flu, especially where there is fever, the Individuality may come out in *dreams of fire, or of danger*. This gives a deeper understanding of the Mental and Emotional symptoms, or the constitutional type, where life is a threat. They must be constantly alert. Think of it, even the air attacks them! "The blighters are everywhere!"

Mercurius

This is not always an easy remedy to spot in its early stages. Like syphilis for which it was routinely used, it is a great imitator. Often I think of it as a *Pulsatilla* that has gone nasty! The key to understanding the syphilitic miasm remedies is *loss of integrity*. Think of the little balls of mercury from a broken thermometer. They scatter into a thousand pieces when touched, and come easily together again if coaxed.

The *Mercurius* patient is very sensitive to *any change of weather*. This will bring on a variety of ailments depending on the patient's vitality. In one it may affect the minor organ of the ear so there is catarrhal build-up and the Individuality of pain *shooting to the right ear from the throat on swallowing, yawning, etc.* In severe cases this pain may shoot even on eating. Since the constitution is run down, these earaches are usually chronic so there is a *foul smelling, even bloody, discharge* through the perforated eardrum.

The acutes of the *Mercurius* patient are 'chronic' in the sense of being recurrent, or simply not clearing up. In this it more resembles *Silicea* as a glandular remedy that is slow to heal. The tonsils easily and continually suppurate especially on the *right side*. The breath is foul smelling. Here the Individuality is *copious salivation*. Constitutionally this flow can be seen in the child with two streams of yellow mucus below the nostrils. In a state of constitutional collapse they will be sensitive to cold but will also *sweat easily*. They will *sweat with pain*, like *Chamomilla* and like *Chamomilla* the smell of discharge may be sour. There will be an easy oozing of sweat all over the body at night. During the day, the hands and feet may be cold but ooze cold sweat like *Silicea*. This is one of those remedies where you must know the Individuality to differentiate clearly.

The acute *Mercurius* symptom picture may also be seen in the digestive system as diarrhoea. Flow is *copious* and *foul smelling* as expected but also *excoriating*. This is the destructive, necrotic syphilitic angle. There may be *much blood* and even *mucus*. *Mercurius* is used in deeper disease such as ulcerative colitis and Crohn's Disease. Its distinct Individuality here is *tenemus even when the rectum has been emptied*. With the diarrhoea come *profuse sweats, especially at night*, and *a creeping chilliness* – both of these increase as vitality decreases.

Such changes in the symptom picture tell us the potency to be used. With sweat and chilliness, or tenemus, we may use the 6th potency and repeat it until vitality increases then end with a 30th potency to deepen the cure on to a preventative level when we are sure the tenemus has gone.

The constitutional symptom picture of *Mercurius* is less common – I suspect because we are fed better and are more aware of our health to allow such collapse. It would suit the weak, sickly type, chilly with cold sweats or night sweats that *stain their clothes yellow*. They will be *prone to colds, mouth ulcers* and *diarrhoea < milk*, or even kidney chills with *burning excoriating urine*.

The personality may be seen more clearly in children. The adults will usually hid their *disgusting filthy habits* although in these days of more open sexuality your morality may be challenged. The *Mercurius* patient is *amoral*. They are tossed by changing fashions because they have no stable inner core. Their self-image is poorly developed and ego boundaries are weak. As a weak personality they are easily led – into the pub to become alcoholics or on to the drug scene. They have no staying power. You may recognise them in the anxious hurried types who cannot be slowed down into contact with society.

SELF TEST

Look through the text for the answers.

1. What is the main fear of *Silicea*?
2. How does the *Silicea* patient react to noise?
3. What might be peculiar about the stool of the *Silicea* patient?
4. How does the *Silicea* patient protect their head?
5. What smells does *Silicea* share with *Hepar sulphuris*?
6. How does the chilliness of the *Hepar sulphuris* patient differ from that of *Mercurius*?
7. Give two peculiarities of the sore throat of the *Hepar sulphuris* patient.
8. How does the essential nature of *Hepar sulphuris* resemble *Rhus toxicodendron*?
9. What is the main modality of *Hepar sulphuris*?
10. Describe the sweat of the *Mercurius* patient.
11. Give three keynotes of the *Mercurius* diarrhoea.
12. Explain the amorality of the *Mercurius* patient.

The Movement of Symptoms According to Hering's Laws of Cure

Homoeopathy is an objective science that studies the Vital Life Force in order to apply its understanding to cure, to heal the sick. All that is visible of the Life Force is its activity. In illness this is the symptoms, so the Homoeopath as Healer studies symptoms.

First the Homoeopath is an **Observer**. We need a clear accurate picture of all the symptoms. As there is only one Vital Force, one organism, so somewhere, somehow, all the symptoms are related. The Homoeopath is looking for **The Total Symptom Picture**.

Next is **interpretation**. What do the symptoms mean? The symptoms will occur on many different levels. On one hand, the patho-physiological processes have a specific and particular interpretation linking the phenomena of the symptoms to what is happening to the physiological processes and to the involved anatomical structures, what the Homoeopath calls the **dysfunction and structural level of disease**. Thus we must isolate what is common to the disease pattern as this contains no, or little, Individuality but by our knowledge of the hierarchy in importance of anatomical systems and types of tissue, we have an idea of how deeply the Vital Force is disturbed – how serious the condition is. This may help our selection of potency.

Sensation, the first level of disease to the Homoeopath, may involve no underlying dysfunction or structural change, or it may be related to underlying change, i.e. pain. The dysfunction level of disease may result in different products or secondary sensations (not discounting pain) and may have further reaching effects such as inefficient metabolism.

Looked at from another angle, the action of the Vital Force is to keep the Whole as intact as possible. In doing this it acts centrifugally to expel disturbance, as symptoms, as far to the outside as it can. It protects its vital core at the expense of the extremities. Thus Constantine Hering's first Law of Cure was **from vital organs to less vital organs**.

It is fundamental to the homoeopathic understanding of disease to see all activity of the Vital Force as an attempt to create cure. Thus 'diseases' such as rheumatism must be understood as expelled to the extremities to protect the most vital part of the circulatory system – the heart. The Homoeopath is not interested in removing symptoms but in initiating the process of cure, to keep the ball rolling in the right direction efficiently with as little aggravation as possible. See Para 2 of the Organon – cure should be gentle.

There is skill in interpreting the movement of symptoms towards cure. It involves knowledge of embryology, the pattern of development of the physiological processes and anatomical structures. If we are to heal naturally we must follow the priorities of the Vital Force. It is not true to say that the homoeopathic remedy aggravates. It increases the movement of the symptoms outwards from the core, protecting the vital processes, from vital organs to less vital organs, using first the natural drains and excretory channels.

Hering's second Law of Cure is **from inside out**. We see it in childhood illnesses which often involve diarrhoea or vomit. Our most common acute, the common cold, involves expulsion, this time of catarrh. The cough is a mechanism that expels violently to keep the airway clear. Vomit and diarrhoea are invaluable in food poisoning. Heat spots and skin disturbances after too acid food show a more metabolic (or **general**) response expelling the excess heat and activity to the outer tube, the skin. Measles is a good example of an illness that is over when the spots come out on the skin. Any damage done by measles is before the spots appear, in the field of complications.

Hering's third Law of Cure takes us beyond the egg stage of the embryo, beyond the tube stage even. Now the organism interacts with gravity and has a sense of **from above downwards**. Hence, where we see this law active, the illnesses are more complicated. On a simple level, pains and discharges move along excretory channels, down the digestive tract, or from the kidneys and bladder down and out, or up from the lungs to the outside – the egg did a somersault in development with the lungs! When we treat skin problems like eczema, the manifestation of disorder comes out to the surface, then proceeds down the trunk or extremities away from the trunk, or centre. Rheumatism that is not caused by injury or repetitive strain likewise moves down from one joint to the one below.

The most useful of Hering's Laws of Cure is the fourth, **in reverse order of occurrence**. The fundamental principle underlying this law is that disease is progressive, if not treated, or if suppressed to deeper levels; thus in earlier years we are healthier. The illnesses of previous years may have been more violent because we had more energy for expulsion, and therefore cure. As time progresses, the organism must find ways to accommodate ill health. If it cannot resolve the disturbance thoroughly, it must make it safe. This is how chronic disease arises from the acute.

The progress of chronic disease is slower. As the disturbance is taken into deeper structures, it takes time to reform then reappear. During this process of slowing down, vitality is locked up, or sapped. The most important practice point for the Homoeopath to note here is that, when the process is reversed through treatment, the Vital Force speeds up again, often becoming more violent as the drains open or the earlier stages of the disease process recur. This is the aggravation of constitutional treatment. A good Homoeopath who has thoroughly taken the case details can usually predict the form the aggravation will take through knowledge of the case, its chosen drains and excretory channels, and Hering's Laws of Cure, and a knowledge of the action of the remedy in different potencies.

ACTIVITY

Knowledge of Hering's Laws of Cure gives us a clear insight into the activity of the Vital Force in health and disease. There can be no substitute here for observation.

Study your own health picture over time. Make a timeline.

A similar study of a few friends, or family, may be eye opening!

EARACHE REPERTORY

Right sided	**bell,** bry, *coloc,* gels, lach, *merc, nux v,* puls, sep,
Lying on right	*lach*
Left sided	acon, lach, nat m, sep
Then right	arn
Pain aching	bell, coloc, lach, nat m, nux v, **puls,** rhus t, sep, sil
boring in	*bell,* coloc, gels, **merc,** nat m, *ruta,* sil
burning	acon, arn, *ars,* bell, bry, *ign,* **merc, nat m**
shooting	*acon, arn, ars,* **bell,** *bry, coloc, hep,* ign, *lach, merc, nat m, nux v,* **puls,** *rhus t,* ruta, sep, *sil*
throbbing	**bell,** *coloc, hep,* lach, merc, nat m, puls, rhus t, sep, *sil*
< blowing nose	hep, puls, sil
< boring with finger	ruta
< chewing	bell, hep, lach, nux v
< from noises	*bell, sil*
< swallowing	**lach,** *merc,* nat m, **nux v**
< in a warm room	*nux v, puls*
Amel warm room	sep
> wrapping up	**hep,** lach, rhus t, *sep*

READING

Theodor Schwenk   Sensitive Chaos   Rudolf Steiner Press

Even if you just look at the pictures you will see patterns of flow, of expansion and resistance, and localisation. It opens the mind to vistas of energy and leads to a deeper understanding of Hahnemann's dynamic plane.

THOUGHT TO PONDER

Now, as diseases are nothing more than alterations in the state of health of the healthy individual which express themselves by morbid signs, and the cure is also only possible by a change to the healthy condition of the state of health of the diseased individual, it is very evident that medicines could never cure diseases if they did not possess the power of altering man's state of health which depends on sensations and functions; indeed, that their curative power must be owing solely to this power they possess of altering man's state of health.

Para 19 The Organon of the Rational Art of Healing
Samuel Hahnemann

LESSON 6   Colds, Coughs and Flus – Winter Ailments

Aims: To study the effect of Vitality on the symptoms produced in a cold.
To study the effect of Vitality on potency selected.
To study further the interaction of the three factors of disease.
To distinguish the levels of defence producing symptoms in a cold.
To explore remedies that arise in colds, coughs and influenza.
To study *Gelsemium* and *Aconite* in greater depth.

Keywords used:
Predisposition
exciting cause
vitality
outer tube
inner tube
middle tube
inflammation
suppuration
minor organ
major organ

The Interaction of Three Factors in Disease

As the order of our studies unfolds, we come to an interesting condition that is acute, local and general at the same time, and 'suppurative'. We have already mentioned Colds, Coughs and Flu in the lessons on Sore Throats and Earache. Here we pay attention to them as an entity in themselves.

To understand the interaction between Predisposition, Exciting Cause and Vitality, I want you to picture five people standing at the bus stop getting soaked. It is bitterly cold with driving rain and the bus is very late; hence the Exciting Cause is < *cold, wet conditions*.

The first person (1) may feel miserable as would anyone in such conditions but he is otherwise unaffected. Cold, wet conditions are not his exciting cause.

The next person (2) is not only miserable, he/she starts to sneeze and shiver as they stand there. They have met their exciting cause. By the time they get home, they have a raging *fever* so need to go to bed with a hot water bottle and a wee toddy. Next morning they know they will be right as rain because they have good vitality and respond quickly and recover quickly. This is the *Belladonna* type and the manifestation is on the **general** level on the first level of the defence mechanism, i.e. fever.

However, (2a) may have just a little less vitality. The organism's defences are further breached so that the Vital Force localises the fever into the lymph glands or the **minor organ**. He/she may develop a sore throat as glands become *inflamed* or a sore ear. When the fever produced would be so high as to be inimitable to life, the person either recovers or dies. So the high fever of *Belladonna* produces delirium and can cause death. Where there is less energy to reach a resolution at that level, the clever Vital Force can side step by localising, even if that means sacrificing the minor organ for the sake of the whole! Those who can produce a generalised fever so quickly are said to have a good level of health, or vitality. Their 'cold' stays at the fever level. When the Vital Force side steps into the minor organ, the level of health is still high but more compromised. Still further compromised, the inflammation will manifest in lymph glands such as the tonsils, thereby activating the next level of defence – *suppuration* or the activity of the white blood cells. This leads into (3).

The third person (3) standing at the bus stop is full of dread because they know what it means. Not only is this their Exciting Cause but they have a tendency to produce colds having a constitutional weakness in the respiratory system (their Predisposition or characteristic pattern) and vitality sufficiently lowered for the disturbance to manifest at the **system** level. Sure enough, but maybe a day or so later, their nose starts to run, they have a bit of a fever or headache or a sore throat, or even earache, but they are generally sluggish. Before the 'cold' has run its course in 1 - 2 weeks, they will go through many boxes of tissues and may need a menthol-eucalyptus lozenge to decongest their tubes. This is the 'cold' proper that we all recognise. It is localised to the upper respiratory system and adjacent structures depending on the individual pattern. Characteristically it produces over-secretion of the mucus membrane lining tissue hence all the catarrh. Individuality is wide ranging from colour of catarrh (white, green, yellow) to the adjacent areas affected (sore throat, earache, headache, sinus) to modalities (< warm rooms, > fresh air, < draughts, < lying down, > hot drinks, < cold drinks) to concomitant symptoms (nausea, dizziness, deafness). Such a broad range of symptoms produces many possible remedies. **You will note that as vitality drops, the symptom picture loses its Individuality, or peaks of clarity.**

The third person standing at the bus stop may be unfortunate in that, if there is even less vitality, the 'cold' does not stop at the upper respiratory but starts to invade the bronchus causing bronchitis, with a little more phlegm, now called expectoration, and perhaps a cough. This might be (3a), temporarily weakened because they have just walked 12 miles, or decorated a room, or up all night swotting for exams – at another time, (3a) might really have the vitality of (2).

When the cough comes by itself, the spasm may be at the (2) level, as in the croup of the *Aconite* patient. Here is an important distinction in how the Homoeopath looks at disease. In (3), the cough is a secondary symptom resulting from the condition of the respiratory system. The croup at (2) is an acute complete in itself with a specific character of accompanying symptoms and a clear individual prognosis.

The individual who produces pneumonia the same night or the following day has a very different type of vitality that is capable of speedy reaction at an inflammatory level but very deeply into the major organ. This is an extreme reaction where the exciting cause may be very virulent or severe and the vitality of the Vital Force is temporarily lowered by another severe cause such as grief. Thus, I have made this into a special category (5) where the **major organ** is disturbed. According to Hering's First Law of Cure, the major organ should be protected and last affected so we will find this situation in the very weak and usually aged (4a), or the very strong. The distinction is important to the Homoeopath because, where the underlying constitution is strong enough to produce such a strong reaction, the potency required is high, chosen to match the speed, and energy, of the Vital Force. Whereas the (3) and (4a) type above is weakened constitutionally and needs built up from a 30th potency, or even a 6th potency, the speedy type has the energy to overcome the situation as quickly as it started so needs at least a 200th potency. You are not advised to treat these as the speed of reaction is so fast that it can move within the hour into totally different remedies.

The fourth person standing at the bus stop may be constitutionally even lower in vitality. Miasmic degeneration may be more active. Usually in a healthy type, or child, the miasm is latent awakening only to the exciting cause as in (2) above. Miasms are taints that stop the Vital Force from reaching optimum health but such is their nature that they continually eat away at health so we see a degenerating pattern with old age. These patterns run in families because they are inherited. Now, depending on the stage of degeneration there is less vitality and such disturbance that the system level dysfunctions and indeed the disturbance is often projected into a secondary system also so the doctor will speak of 'chronic disease'. This type of case is recognised because the susceptibility of the Vital Force is **activated by the modality,** rather than the exciting cause, and the symptoms produced seem to ooze out at the system level, rather than respond with vitality as an acute. His is the *disease process.* So, in this case, the Vital Force is further weakened by its modalities of *cold, wet.*

The healthier type of (4) may attempt an acute but here it is thrown out at a general level as in flu, where the whole organism may be disturbed by malaise. With their lowered vitality, it takes a few days to produce the symptoms. Hence they feel under the weather for a few days, their limbs start to ache as the inflammatory processes are kept to the periphery in the extremities, in connective tissue of muscles. The sluggishness is accompanied by fatigue and stupor, cannot think or concentrate, as toxins invade the blood stream affecting the brain and nervous system. In the general malaise, they lose their appetite. Individual difference may involve headache, chills up and down the spine or chilly feet and hands, catarrh in the upper respiratory system, cough. It may be complicated with bronchitis or pleurisy if prolonged.

A less healthy type (4a), on exposure to the modality, may quickly produce bronchitis, or even pleurisy or pneumonia in an older person. The last two are very different from the pneumonia of (5). Here there is too little vitality. Many old people die from pneumonia rather than the chronic disease for which they are being treated. They are afflicted but have no vitality to correct the disturbance.

In treating type (4), you need to lower the potency of the remedy used and work slowly building up the vitality. Remedies will need to be repeated and changed as vitality increases. Real improvement will only occur when there is the vitality, or reactive space, to respond to the constitutional remedy. Indeed, they may need the constitutional remedy rather than the acute remedy but, either way, constitutional treatment is required at the end of the 'acute' to create better health. However, remember they have less vitality so constitutional treatment is not the 1M and 10M potencies. If you look at the case, you will see few **general** symptoms and many, many symptoms of a **particular** nature, of dysfunction and even structural change. Many symptoms will be the **products** of system dysfunction, e.g. catarrh. Unfortunately, most of our work today as Homoeopaths lies with types (3) and (4).

In summary

There are several keys in the above to the Homoeopath. Without the exciting cause, there would be no illness. Likewise it is the underlying predisposition that creates the susceptibility to the exciting cause and the individual differences of the constitution that tell us the essential nature and susceptibility of this Vital Force. Of great importance is the lowered vitality. This is tricky because some predispositions (constitutions) are weaker than others so do allow disturbance into deeper levels of defence (i.e. 4).

Before anyone can become ill they need three things – the **predisposition** that determines the character of the illness, **to meet the exciting cause** or weakness of the Vital Force, and **lowered vitality**. The speed of the reaction to the exciting cause is related to the vitality of the person at that time and to their general quality of health. Category 2 above is the child or very healthy *Belladonna* type who can produce an inflammatory reaction. (2a) is the same constitutional type with lowered vitality. Category 3 is usually the less healthy Vital Force of the *Pulsatilla* or *Bryonia*, who can nevertheless produce an acute in the minor organ in the most vital type of this category – as opposed to (2a) this is usually suppurative rather than inflammatory. Both remedies may produce some inflammation but deeper, into the system level. They are more noted for producing over-secretion of mucus in the upper respiratory system, i.e. in the inner tube and with the second level of defence, suppuration. Category 4 responds generally at the second level of defence with the deeper disturbance of the flu as a more general disturbance. The 5th category as already explained is a strongest Vital Force but severely stressed either by an extreme exciting cause or temporary steep drop in vitality, often both.

The speed of development tells the Homoeopath the type of remedy and the potency to use to restore health in the speediest time.

This is so important to the treatment of acutes that a summarising table might be in order, but first an exercise.

> **EXERCISE**
>
> Study your own cold symptoms paying attention to symptoms of Individuality, to exciting causes and modalities. How does your vitality drop?
>
> Into which category in the table on the next page would you place your symptoms?

Table summarising interaction of Predisposition, Exciting Cause and Vitality

Category	Level of defence	Symptoms	Potency*	Comments
1	None – healthy			
2	**General** Fever Reaction to Exciting Cause	Heat, throbbing pains, sweat, maybe delirium if severe. Redness on skin as symptoms expelled to outside – *to outer tube.*	30th - 200th depending on severity, even 1M	Speed of onset is very fast. Recovery, or death, is just as fast.
2a	**Minor Organ** Inflammation Reaction to Exciting Cause	Heat, throbbing pains, redness of part, swelling.	30th - 200th depending on severity	Speed of onset is very fast. Response to remedy should be just as fast.
3	**Upper Respiratory** Low fever and Suppuration (production of catarrh/mucus) To **minor organ** inflammatory low grade to suppuration. Reaction to Exciting Cause + Lowered Vitality	Catarrhal discharge becoming drier or more copious so stitching pain or dull ache with congestion Inner *tube affected.*	Repeat 6th if not severe or if a child – hourly. 30th if in 2nd stage (e.g. drier stage) or general symptoms such as chill – repeat after 3-6 hourly in higher potency if needed.	Onset is slow – maybe 12-24 hours or more if less vitality. Repetition of dose may be needed to push symptoms on if there is sluggishness. Change the remedy or potency as energy increases.
3a	**Respiratory** More suppurative becoming congested or drier. Can become bronchitis, pleurisy even but rare. Reaction to Exciting Cause + Lowered Vitality	This is slow expansion deeper into the **respir. system** indicating lower vitality.	Lower potency 6-30th and/or different acute remedy is needed and HELP from expert to match the speed of the potency to the needs of the Vital Force. DO NOT REPEAT THE SAME POTENCY	What is needed to raise Vitality? What might support the system E.g. steaming, postural drainage, total rest, Vitamin C, diets to build up energy. Case management to build up the patient.
4	**General** Influenza May be Exciting Cause but Modality increasingly important. Predisposition in weaker constitution.	Fever. Aching in connective tissue Middle *tube affected – could be heart in rheumatic fever.* Dopey, often catarrh and either sweat or dryness. Dull red if coloured.	30th – depending on severity. If there is not enough resolution within 12 – 24 hours repeat the 30th potency. Constitutional treatment should follow.	This takes several days to get going and there is a general malaise in the build-up.
4a	**Systemic Disease**	Weakened respiratory system is easily afflicted by exposure to modality, e.g. cold, damp to produce chronic bronchitis.	Repeat doses of 6th potency may be needed. Take care on raising to 30th that you activate the miasm and increase severity of symptoms. Needs expert and constitutional treatment.	The weakened Vital Force is looking for expression, which is the only way to better health. These are good cases to use 9th and 12th potencies! Go slowly so as to strengthen vitality rather than use it up.

Category	Level of defence	Symptoms	Potency*	Comments
5	**Major Organ** Inflammatory Reaction to Exciting Cause + Lowered Vitality. Strong constitution.	Heat, severe pain, emotional response such as anguish or fear.	200th - 1m depending on severity and other symptoms. Use lower potency if there is much thick expectoration to shift or patient is very weak.	You need expert help for this one.

* The potency suggestions can only be generalised. Each case is unique.

Winter Ailments

I choose this term specifically because it alludes to a phenomenon with which we are so familiar that we should not accept and pass it without questioning how it fits into our understanding of the disease process. We expect colds in the winter. Indeed some of us think it is normal to have a dose of influenza in the winter. To what are we alluding?

In our climate the cold, wet of winter is an exciting cause to many of us. Continual exposure often means that our vitality drops in the winter so we are more prone to minor aberrations of health. There is less sun in winter to manufacture Vitamin D. Alas, we do not have the excuse of our ancestors that there is less fruit and fresh vegetables in Nature's quiet phase. We spend more time indoors, in poorly ventilated hot trains or buses, in artificially heated offices. We are herded together in unhygienic situations. There is the continual stress to the Vital Force of changing from overheated to cold, wet environments. Such conditions would lower anyone's Vital Force along the lines of maintaining causes, but there is something else.

Many of us in the west of Europe, especially in Scotland and Ireland, have an underlying miasm of tuberculosis developed from our ancestors' exposure in the industrial age to crowded, closed-in living quarters and factories and poor nutrition. The miasms give us the underlying predisposition to disease. In the tubercular miasm, a main weakness is cold, wet conditions as the exciting cause. The weak location is of course the respiratory system that first meets the 'cold wet' internally and the level of defence is usually the suppurative through the white blood cells, the lymph system and glands. These two factors present the syndrome we know as colds.

> **EXERCISE**
>
> Research your family history to determine the role of tuberculosis and respiratory disease in your immediate ancestors.
>
> Study the similarity between 'cold' symptoms in different family members. Pay attention to individuality, modality and exciting cause.
>
> Now, if possible, share this with class members to study the difference in non-family members.

Coughs

Coughs are simply a spasm of the bronchi and intercostal muscles, sometimes the diaphragm, in which air is forced out of the lungs with such force as to clear the air passages and expel solid or liquid matter.

COUGH! Which muscles are you using? How did you start to cough?

The trachea and bronchi are ringed with cartilage to keep them open. The lining is mucus membrane with secretory cells producing the moist environment plus special cells with little cilia (hairs) that sweep out the debris. In the smoker these are paralysed by the tobacco so mucus builds up but in the morning before that first cigarette they come alive and start to clear out the mucus giving rise to the familiar smoker's cough!

The cough is a defensive mechanism to keep the airway clear. When it becomes a problem it is either because there is excessive spasm as in asthma or whooping cough, or there is excess mucus to clear as in a cold. In some types of cold the lining mucus membrane becomes dry and congested so either the mucus is tenacious and thick requiring the cough to expel it or the dryness itself creates irritation. Usually the cough occurs as part of another illness. I have given some indication above as to treatment when it is part of an illness. Here I will look only at cough, as in category (2a) or at the start of category (3).

Now we need to describe the cough. In category (2a) it may arise from the dryness of the inflammatory processes. In (3) it may occur as mucus is secreted and needs to be externalised. Where it occurs as an acute in itself, as in croup, it is often spasmodic. Once again each case is unique and this is only a broad generalisation. It is useful in its guide to potency.

Dry cough may be inflammatory as in *Aconite, Belladonna, Ferrum Phosphoricum*. It will then come with a fever and redness of the pharynx plus other individual symptoms of these remedies.

Belladonna   tickles and is sensitive to movement. There are violent paroxysms as if the head would burst that often end in sneezing. The patient is dry and hot, especially about the head. The artery leading to the head (*carotid*) may throb visibly. They are worse eating and drinking warm things. Where the dry cough is not inflammatory but congested locally, *Bryonia* is a common remedy.

Bryonia   This illness starts with copious mucus then there is a dry stage representing lack of action. There may be a stitch-like pain on any movement as the dry parts stick. Thus, they are seen to hold the throat, or the chest, as they cough to try to prevent movement. The cough is described as hard – as the illness progresses the whole chest is involved. Then deep breathing hurts them as it moves the whole chest down to the lungs. They are better for long drinks and worse for heat that dries the tubes further. Like *Belladonna* each cough can explode into the head but in *Bryonia* only if the sinuses are also congested.

Wheezing, rattling cough means copious mucus. It may be in the bronchi or much deeper into the lungs themselves. This is a deeper level of defence action producing excessive mucus. *Bryonia* is often the remedy if other symptoms agree, e.g. yellowish catarrh and great thirst (Concomitant). *Pulsatilla* occurs in mucusy colds with copious white catarrh, but whilst it may reach into the minor organ of the ear, it goes up to the sinus of the head rather than to the lungs or bronchus (Location). Deeper into the lungs we start to think of remedies of even weaker states such as *Antimonium tartaricum* or *Arsenicum*.

On the other hand, *Phosphorus* fits all levels of vitality and is recognisable by its symptom of < talking or < any breath of cold air (modality). Its sensation is a tickle which often appears when they are on the telephone because they are talking and also because of the electromagnetism in the telephone itself – another of *Phosphorus* modalities. Because such coughs are a sign of weakened vitality, they often need expert care and attention. This same weakness often means the symptom picture is undistinguished so we must look for Individuality in such as Time, Location, Sensation, Modality and Concomitant.

Spasmodic coughs occur more commonly on their own after exposure to cold, dry conditions as in *Hepar sulphuris, Causticum, Ipecacuanha, Bryonia, Nux vomica, Spongia* and *Drosera*.

Ipecacuanha incessant < every breath. They suffocate as they retch with spasm then eventually vomit mucus. They may be red or blue in the face. The child stiffens all over with the spasms.

Nux vomica is dry with gagging and retching (reversed peristalsis) because they are over-sensitive and sensation in trachea starts off spasm in the digestive tract. The cough therefore is worse eating and drinking. They may have a bursting headache as they cough because the muscles are so tense. The whole situation starts after exposure to cold, dry conditions. Although chilly, they overheat easily when covered but rapidly cool when uncovered.

EXERCISE

Here is a comparison of three cough remedies. Continue the table adding other remedies you have studied. Pay attention to **Time, Location, Sensation, Modality and Concomitant** to enable differentiation.

	Aconite	*Spongia*	*Drosera*
Time	< after midnight < until 3am	< day & night < after rising	< after midnight < evening < 3am
Exciting cause	< COLD, DRY < open air < draught of cold air change of temperature from excitement from fright	< Cold, dry FROM EXCITEMENT from exertion	 after measles
Type	BARKING LOUD	BARKING day and night	BARKING on becoming warm
Sensation	Burning in larynx	Burning in larynx Constriction of larynx	Constriction of larynx with convulsions Crawling in larynx As if a feather
Modalities	< deep breathing esp. expiration < after drinking < eating < lying on side Grasps throat	< bending backwards > after drinking > EATING	< deep breathing esp. expiration < after drinking < eating Grasps throat

Influenza

This is an interesting illness from a homoeopathic point of view. As a Winter Ailment, it is most prevalent when the weather changes. However, it strikes so many it is truly epidemic – people catch it! It spreads rapidly through offices in days. In my early days as a Homoeopath I spent ages talking students and patients out of the 'germ theory' of disease knowing that Pasteur himself agreed with me that it was the terrain that determined the weed that grew. As a gardener, I forgot how virulent weeds are and that should have challenged my theory. However, there is more to it than this. Influenza is a relatively recent disease, i.e. centuries old.

If the Homoeopath has four types of acute disease – **sporadic, endemic, epidemic** and **contagious** – then influenza falls into the epidemic category when the population is prey to a virulent antagonist because vitality is lowered as after disasters. In studying the flu over 15 years at least, I have seen them linked to national events and to seasonal stress such as Christmas, and especially after national events such as financial dips. The Great Flu that killed more than the Great War would fit into this frame. However, in an epidemic not everyone becomes ill. Indeed, even the Great Plague killed only 40% of the population. Why are some 'too healthy' to catch it? Even in an epidemic, when vitality is lowered and the cause is virulent, you must have predisposition. Some are more prone to flu. Some know they will escape, or escape lightly, if their vitality is high. To catch flu you need the taint of the tubercular miasm. Now look at which populations are most likely to be devastated by flu each year. It is a disease of civilised, industrialised populations. It is not a rural disease. It has increased in incidence and come worldwide in wave after wave with **geographical mobility**. It could fit into Hahnemann's *contagious* category. Major characteristics of the tubercular miasm are *civilised, geographical mobility, respiratory weakness, < cold and wet, disappointment.* As a miasm, it is often called **pseudo-psora** because it is psora at a deeper level where its main affinity is for the inner tube, especially the respiratory system. Influenza strikes at so many people because they have a weaker constitution; pseudo-psora disturbed the Vital Force more deeply than psora. The main remedies of influenza also cover the tubercular miasm.

Now we can see category (4) when it is healthy enough to throw out an acute albeit on the general level. And we should be able to understand why one of the main characteristics of flu is *aches and pains* as it affects the *middle tube*, i.e. it strikes deeper than most acutes. So the 30th potency is the most usual with which to tackle influenza. Also needed is constitutional treatment if not also convalescence to build up a better health profile.

Remedies

Arnica   has aching, sore, *bruised* muscles. They feel pressure sitting or lying so are *restless. The bed feels hard. Parts lain on feel chilly.* They are mentally prostrate and dopey, falling asleep when answering your questions. They are morose, grumpy and say nothing is wrong – *leave me alone.* There may be digestive symptoms of vomit and nausea at the start leading to great dullness of consciousness.

Pyrogen   Unfortunately, this is becoming more common. *There are intense generalised aches and pains all over, as in Arnica. They are also restless and sensitive to pressure. More individually they are* sensitive to draughts –> sneezing. *Mentally they are so overactive they become* talkative *or even delirious – their limbs are all over the bed (as in Baptisia). Like Arsenicum they are anxious and sip frequent small quantities of water. They have a congestive headache at the temples that is better for pressure.*

Bryonia   is slow to develop. There is great muscular *exhaustion especially in the thighs. < right side.* As they become increasingly dopey, the respiratory system is affected. As this dries there is a *cough on deep inspiration.* They drink *great draughts of water.* They are *touchy* and irritable. In their distress, they will be *anxious about their work;* in delirium, they will *want to go home.* As they become more congested there will be a *bursting headache on coughing.* Even the *eyeballs will be painful on movement.*

Gelsemium Once again there is a slow onset after exposure to *cold, wet* conditions. There are *weak heavy muscles*. The heaviness is such that they *cannot keep their eyes open*. They want to be left alone, are prostrate, *indifferent*, and *answer slowly* if at all. As the illness progresses their *limbs will tremble* so they cannot control them. There will be *chills especially on the spine*. They are described as having *tight throats and empty heads*. Eventually the nervous system is so affected they *see double*.

Never Been Well Since Flu

Unfortunately, this is a common phenomenon especially in the last few years. Indeed, it arises as many stagger from one bout to another, have a respite in summer then relapse again at the first chill of winter. Although many are labelled as having ME, it is not as drastic as that. The Vital Force simply does not have the vitality to recover so needs built up and prodded gently and more frequently till energy is restored, then constitutional treatment is necessary.

Unfortunately, two things conspire against us as Homoeopaths. Convalescence to allow vitality to be restored is not taken seriously as the patient rushes back to work or into the social whirl; and similarly, patients do not allow us to get to the constitutional stage of the treatment because their concept of health is frequently not as high as our's.

Remedies

Gelsemium

This plant brings forth yellow flowers *in the winter*. It is the Winter Jasmine. It is a sensitive plant that sends out tendrils to cling to others as it climbs so it comes as no surprise that it is a remedy of nervous temperaments.

We use it in First Aid for shock, for ailments from bad news. It is also one of our remedies of anticipation that occurs before events such as exams. In both these situations they *tremble at the knees* and may rush to the toilet with *diarrhoea*. They are *benumbed*. It may be a remedy of panic attacks when there are palpitations with nervous excitability. In extreme cases, there is a *fear to move in case the heart stops*. We do not need to allow it to get to this extreme fear to get the sense of holding back on the patient's behalf, for fear that something will happen. They may feel a flutter of excitement or restless that prevents action.

It is commonly seen as a remedy of chill which affects the nervous system. The anxiety may be characterised by a *chill or shiver down the spine*. Cold, wet conditions will bring a runny nose that moves into the glands. It is one of the remedies that will produce yellow diarrhoea as a reaction to chill. At this level, they will recover quickly even without treatment. With less vitality, they are prone to influenza distinguished by *weakness, heaviness and trembling*. As such, it is a remedy of congestion and lack of flow. It is the lack of fluid absorption at the muscular level that gives the symptom of heaviness and weakness (as after heavy and unusual exercise). *The trembling arises when they try to move*. As the congestion continues they become dull and drowsy, so *they cannot think*. Ultimately this is a remedy of paralysis, of progressive *locomotor ataxia*. In the flu, they cannot raise their head. They have no energy to open their eyes. There are chills down the spine.

The remedy affects cerebro-spinal fluid balance so there are severe *heavy* congestive *headaches that are better from urinating*. It is no surprise to find they are *thirstless*, or *worse before thunderstorms*. This last seems to give rise to pressure on the head! Depression is their response to the world. They cut off and want to be left alone. This is cutting out stimulation moving inwards, away from the 'bad world'. *Numbness* is a common feature and this too is dulling the senses to the external world. Yet, initially, their response to the trembling is a *desire to be held tight* to stop the trembling. Thus, we see the remedy opposites here – first a desire to cling, then to move away from the source of distress into their inner world. This last corresponds with the paralysis state.

In its final stage, the *Gelsemium* patient is *apathetic and indifferent*. They *cannot grasp thoughts* but *answer slowly*. The limbs are heavy and *lack co-ordination*. With palpitation and possibly panic attacks, we often see this symptoms picture at menopause, or even before menses. As a remedy of the old person, we might add chills up and down the spine, emptiness at the epigastrium and yellow diarrhoea, and anticipatory anxiety. There may be vertigo with a fear of falling.

Aconite

This is a remedy of the very healthiest who react rapidly to their exciting cause. In *cold dry conditions*, they may rapidly develop a fever that is accompanied by a *restless anxiety*. In the highest fevers there may be restless sleep, *tossing and turning* with bad dreams, even delirium. At worst, they will *fear they might die*. Usually they are better by morning.

When it strikes deeper into the respiratory system, we might see sneezing even as they stand at the bus stop. If this develops into fever, once again, it may be gone by morning. However, there is a possibility it may affect the minor organ of the ear. Here we see its individuality in that it is the *left* ear. There is characteristic redness, heat and throbbing pain. More individualistic is the *great sensitivity to noise*. It is a simple acute that will respond to applications of heat, or a dose of *Aconite 6* or *30*. *Aconite* seldom goes deeper into the respiratory system.

We often say it is useful at the start of troubles! This really refers to the fact it is only a remedy of inflammation and not deeper stages of suppuration. J. T. Kent says *it comes and goes like a great storm*. However, it can be found in pneumonia, *of the apex of the left lung*. Here it is in the inflammatory stage. The chest feels *hot*. There is a *tingling* in the chest after coughing. Remember such a patient has very strong vitality so will react rapidly to a high potency, 30th or 1M.

More common is croup. In the first stages of the tubercular miasm, there is a tendency to high fevers, especially in children. It is this level of energy that will respond with croup on exposure to cold dry conditions. Now there is fear because there is a very real possibility of dying. They are worse whenever they attempt to breathe in. You may see pallor and cold drenching sweat but the most individual symptom of the croup is that it starts at midnight in bed. It is in serious disturbances such as croup and pneumonia that you will see the individualistic symptoms of *sweats on uncovered parts* and *thirst* when everything *tastes bitter except water*.

Although it presents in early inflammation, *Aconite* is a nervous system remedy. We have seen the anxiety above. We say the **sensation** of *Aconite* is a tingle and can see that in the chest symptoms above. The pains of *Aconite* are often *tearing* where nerves are involved. All these symptoms come together in *trigeminal neuralgia* brought on by exposure to cold dry conditions and, of course, on the *left* side. We will also see *Aconite* as a remedy in toothache where the pains are tearing, < cold and give rise to severe anxiety.

On an acute level, the main nervous symptom is *fear*. *Aconite* is a remedy of terror, < midnight – the witching hour. It is an irrational, life threatening fear. When they fear to die at a certain hour, Kent would put the clock back giving the remedy time to work because they will die. It is remedy of paralysing fear. They lose the use of their eyes if they see something awful. They lose the use of their ears if they hear something awful. The hand that offends is paralysed. This is a primitive fear. *Aconite* restores the use of the eyes, ears or hand! In *fright,* it is the remedy of pallor, cold drenching sweat, *pupils drawn into pinpricks,* involuntary urination, rapid bounding pulse. It is a remedy for retention of urine in the newborn child. You will never fail to recognise the *Aconite* patient if you have a sense of the fearfulness that lies beneath their ruddy glow.

In Homoeopathy, these mental and emotional symptoms give us the complete picture – the **Total Symptom Picture**.

SHORT REPERTORY OF COLDS AND COUGHS

Nose
- coryza
  - starts right side — arn, **ars**, **bell**, *bry*, **merc**, **puls**
  - starts left side — acon, *lach*, sep, **sil**
- **Catarrh** left side — lach, sep
  - \> open air — *bry*, **puls**
  - < cold weather — ars
  - dry chronic — *nat m*, **sil**
  - offensive — ars, bell, **hep**, *lach*, led, **merc**, nux v, **puls**, *sep*, **sil**
  - extending to front sinus — ars, bry, **merc**, *nux v*, *puls*, **sil**
  - post nasal — acon, bry, **nat m**, *rhus t*, sep, *sil*
  - bloody — acon, **ars**, **bell**, bry, gels, **hep**, *lach*, led, **merc**, *nat m*, nux v, puls, rhus t, sep, sil
  - excoriating — **ars**, *gels*, *hep*, ign, *lach*, **merc**, nat m, **nux v**, puls, *rhus t*, sep, *sil*
  - dry hard — ars, *bry*, *lach*, merc, **sep**, **sil**
  - purulent — ars, bell, **hep**, ign, *lach*, led, **merc**, *nat m*, nux v, **puls**, *rhus t*, *sep*, **sil**
  - scabs inside — ars, bry, *hep*, lach, merc, nat m, nux v, *puls*, **sep**, *sil*
  - viscid — ars, hep, *sep*, *sil*
  - watery — **ars**, bell, *bry*, coloc, gels, ign, lach, **merc**, *nat m*, **nux v**, puls, sep, *sil*
  - yellow — acon, *ars*, **hep**, *lach*, *nat m*, **puls**, rhus t, sep, *sil*
  - green — arn, ars, *bry*, cimic, hep, led, **merc**, nux v, **puls**, *rhus t*, **sep**, *sil*
- **Glands**
  - swollen tonsils — **bell**, *gels*, **hep**, ign, *lach*, led, *merc*, nux v, puls, sep, **sil**
  - suppurated tonsils — *bell*, **hep**, ign, *lach*, **merc**, *sep*, **sil**
- **Cough**
  - barking — **acon, bell, hep,** merc
  - On breathing deeply — *acon*, arn, ars, **bell**, **bry**, **hep**, lach, *merc*, nat m, *puls*, *rhus t*, sep, sil
  - With brining in the chest — led
  - With burning in the throat — ars, bell
  - Choking — ars, *hep*, *lach*, *puls*, **rhus t**, *sep*, sil
  - On becoming cold — arn, **ars**, *bry*, **hep**, *lach*, **nux v**, **rhus t**, **sil**
  - Going from warmth to cold — *acon, nux v,* sep
  - Croupy — **acon**, *ars*, *bell*, *gels*, **hep**, *lach*, ruta
- Dry, in the morning — *ars*, bry, hep, ign, nux v, *rhus t*, sep, sil
- Dry, at night, loose in day — acon, ars, bry, *hep*, lach, merc, nux v, *puls*, sil
- Dry, < lying down — *puls*
- Dry, with expectoration morning only — bell, *bry*, *hep*, led, *nat m*, nux v, **puls**, *sep*, *sil*
- Dry, with fever — **acon**, *arn*, *ars*, bell, **bry**, hep, ign, lach, **nat m**, **nux v**, puls, rhus t, sep
- Dry, from tickling in larynx — *bell*, cimic, coloc, *lach*, led, *nat m*, nux v, **puls**, *sep*
- From dry air passages — lach, merc, *puls*
- From dry larynx — bell, bry, lach, *nux v*, *puls*, rhus t
- From dry spot — cimic
- From dry trachea — *puls*
- < eating — acon, arn, *ars*, bell, *bry*, hep, lach, nat m, **nux v**, puls, rhus t, ruta, *sep*, sil
- Hacking, on lying down — *ars*, bry, *ign*, lach, nat m, rhus t, sep, sil
- Hacking, from raw larynx — bry, sil
- Hacking, tickling in larynx — acon, **ars**, *bry*, **lach**, **nat m**, rhus t, sep, sil

Hollow,	*acon,* **bell**, bry, hep, *ign,* lach, led, merc, nux v, sil
On inspiration	acon, bell, *hep,* lach, *puls*
< the more one coughs	*bell,* **ign**
on laughing	ars, bry, lach, rhus t, sil
< lying down	acon, *arn,* ars, bell, *bry,* hep, ign, *lach,* merc, nat m, nux v, **puls**, *rhus t,* sep, sil
< motion	arn, *ars,* bell, *bry,* lach, led, merc, nat m, *nux v,* sep, *sil*
nervous cough	*hep, ign,* lach, nux v
racking	*arn,* ars, **bell, bry, ign,** *lach,* led, **merc**, nat m, **nux v, puls**, *rhus t, sep, sil*
racking, < evening	led, nat m, *puls,* rhus t
racking, on rising from bed	acon, ars, bry, ign, **lach**, sep
racking, on going to sleep	arn, *hep,* ign, **lach**, merc, sep
Wakes from sleep	acon, arn, *ars,* bell, hep, *lach,* merc, *rhus t, sep*
Ends in sneezing	*bell,* bry, hep
Spasmodic	acon, *ars,* **bell, bry,** coloc, *gels, hep, ign, lach, led, merc, nat m,* **nux v, puls,** *rhus t,* **sep,** sil
<in a warm room	acon, arn, ars, *bry,* **puls**
<in wind	*acon,* **hep**, sep

PRACTICE POINT

Students and practitioners may be quite frustrated at this point because the rubrics and the remedies contained in these repertories are very limited! This should emphasise certain points:

1. There are over 2000 homoeopathic remedies and I have included only those in your First Aid box. If they are used in a low enough potency there will be enough of an overlap for you to get results.

2. If you look at the entries, the same remedies keep appearing so you need to discriminate carefully the value of each remedy under the chosen rubric. Some homoeopathic remedies have a very wide field of action but, although they appear in the rubric, may not be the most efficient remedy in this condition.

3. You need to choose the rubrics very carefully to include *Individuality*. I have included many rubrics to demonstrate the precision of the Homoeopath in selecting a remedy. You will also recognise the need to describe the symptom very clearly.

Hopefully this will give a deeper understanding of how your Homoeopath is asking you to describe your symptoms, and may explain the frustration of the Homoeopath on the other end of the telephone when you ask for help in an acute. The detail needed is exacting.

It is very difficult to do harm with Homoeopathy especially if you remember the two golden rules:

- never repeat the remedy
- never go down in potency.

> You can repeat the 6th potency up to three times but do not persist if there is no change in the symptoms – **the remedy is not similar enough to the symptom picture**. Remember, if there is no change, take the case again. If there is change then relapse, watch the distance between the relapse. If the gap is becoming less, you need to increase the potency, or find a better fit remedy. If the gap is lengthening, that is good. You can repeat the remedy as long as the gap continues to lengthen.
>
> Use only one dose of the 30th potency and look for the symptoms to change according to Hering's Laws of Cure. Repeat only if the symptoms relapse and you are sure of your remedy. If in any doubt contact your Homoeopath. If you are under treatment from a Homoeopath, they should know that you are using 30th potencies as most remedies will interact with their constitutional treatment.

Putting it all together

Now you have a little bit of repertory, let us work on a few cases. My comments and answers follow, so you may want to cover up part of the page until you have worked it out for yourself.

1. After being out in a sharp cold spell during the day, the old lady has started to sneeze violently this evening. Copious fluid running from her nose started on the left side. She is very restless so cannot get to sleep. You might be surprised to find this remedy in an old lady, but why not?

    So, you have the exciting cause of < cold exposure. From the repertory above you can find coryza starting on the left side. That will give your 4 remedies. You need knowledge of previous *Materia Medica* to tell you which of these four have the exciting cause of exposure to cold and you have the characteristic restless to confirm you choice of *Aconite*. Now, as to potency, although old this old lady has good vitality because it started within hours of exposure and the symptoms are at the first level of response with no complications in the respiratory system. Thus a 6th potency will no doubt do the trick. You might have considered a 30th potency if her defence responses were blunted by old age or drug taking but see how quickly she has responded.

2. Again after exposure to a cold dry snap, the child has developed a dry cough when he breathes deeply. The following morning you discover yellow purulent catarrh. The patient is very chilly and cough is worse on the slightest uncovering.

    Here you have a line of remedies with dry cough and expectoration in the morning only. The yellow catarrh rubric only gets rid of *Nux vomica*. If you know your *Materia Medica* the dryness of the cold snap may dispose of a few more remedies. However, one of the chilliest remedies in the *Materia Medica* has the keynote < uncovering. When it is also a common remedy in dry coughs you have no hesitating in prescribing *Hepar sulphuris calcarea* this time in the 30th potency because the purulent catarrh shows a deeper penetration of the disturbance.

3. After exposure to wet weather, this child has a spasmodic cough that is worse on entering a warm room or on lying down. When I tell you the child is whiny you will have no problem finding a remedy but what about potency?

Aconite, Arsenicum, Bryonia and *Pulsatilla* are the four remedies with spasmodic cough < on entering a warm room and < lying down. *Aconite* is < cold, dry conditions so is less well indicated (but do not dismiss it on a negative argument). However, the *Pulsatilla* child is notoriously whiny. What potency? There are no complications or indications that the exposure has affected deeply. My choice between the 6th and the 30th potency might depend on how quickly the child took to develop the symptoms. If they developed after hours do not waste a 30th potency but use the 6th; but if it took 24 hours use a single dose of the 30th potency as slower vitality is indicated. [1]

4. This patient has much yellow catarrh forming hard crusts < on the left side. There is coloured matter on the tonsils showing they are suppurating. The breath is foul. Some blood is present on the catarrh, and this shy child has a nervous cough as you ask to see the tonsils.

   This time there is no noted exciting cause. The Individuality is hard crust, left side, yellow, bloody and tonsils suppurating. The repertory above brings you down to *Arsenicum, Lachesis, Sepia* and *Silicea*. The suppurating tonsils may exclude *Arsenicum*. It is the nervous cough that points to *Lachesis* which is renowned for its foul breath. As to potency, the suppurating state points to the deep disturbance, the second level of defence, that needs the 30th potency. Single dose should do the trick.

5. You have never heard a hollow cough before. This one is worse breathing in since exposure to cold wet weather. One cough starts off paroxysms as if the man would never stop. When he coughs he also complains of the throat burning.

   Hollow cough on inspiration has three remedies: *Belladonna, Hepar sulphuris calcarea* and *Lachesis*. One cough starts another has only *Belladonna* which is confirmed in the rubric *burning in the throat on coughing*. The exciting cause of cold wet would not favour *Hepar Sulphuris calcarea* and your knowledge of *Materia Medica* should tell you that *Lachesis* is often associated with burning as a sensation and the larynx as an affinity. So *Belladonna* repertorises but why choose it? It has a higher grade of symptom that either of the other two in the hollow cough rubric. Also, it appears in italics in the rubric *one cough starts a paroxysm*. In a child the 6th potency might have been sufficient but since this is an adult, and it sounds like severe inflammation, I would choose one dose of the 30th potency of *Belladonna*.

The more repertorising you do the more familiar you will become with the *Materia Medica* and with using the philosophy to select your remedy.

---

[1] Homoeopathy is full of contradictions. Elsewhere, I will suggest the 6th potency because there is less vitality to respond to it. With children and in acute cases, the disturbance is seldom deep so again only need a little stimulation with the remedy.

READINGS

Ethel Douglas Hume   Bechamp or Pasteur   Pub C. W. Daniel Co Ltd
Also called "Pasteur Exposed" and published by Bookreal, Australia

> *An astonishing book on the history of germ theory purporting to show that 'vaccination far from saving millions of lives has cost millions'.*

Rene Dubois   The Mirage of Health   Rutgers University Press

> *'An exceptional book – plain, lucid, elegant, lively. It draws its facts and illustrations not only from the corpus of medicine but from authors from Lao-tzu to Proust. It is logical and persuasive ... a confession of faith and humility by a great scientist.' – Lancet. What more could I add? This man is a great thinker.*

THOUGHT TO PONDER

> *The inimical forces, partly psychical, partly physical, to which our terrestrial existence is exposed, which are termed morbific obnoxious agents, do not possess the power of morbidly deranging the health of man unconditionally; but we are made ill by them only when our organism is sufficiently disposed and susceptible to the attack of the morbific cause that may be present, and to be altered in its health, deranged and made to undergo abnormal sensations and functions – hence they do not produce disease in every one nor at all times.*
>
> Para 31, The Organon of the Rational Art of Healing
> Samuel Hahnemann

LESSON 7   The Digestive System

Aims: To discuss a homoeopathic approach to digestive disturbances.
To demonstrate the difference between the Maintaining and Exciting Cause in digestive disturbances.
To study the relationship between the anatomy and physiology and the symptom picture.
To study acute disturbance in a system.
To study the relationship between repetition of the dose and the symptom picture.
To learn criteria related to increasing the potency.
To study *Arsenicum, Ipecacuanha, Ignatia, Colocynth.*

Keywords used:
Maintaining cause
exciting cause
susceptibility
individuality
symptom picture

the inner tube
dysfunction in a system
affinity
the outer tube

modalities
essence
total symptom picture
indicating symptoms

Digestive Disturbance is a Common Occurrence

Disturbance in the digestive system is common. Who has not had a sore tummy? This is a key location for exposure to the outer world, the not-me world, so it is a prime site for rapid readjustments!

The skin is the outer tube; the digestive system is part of the inner tube. The movement of symptoms is out to the edge of the pond, the skin. With excess energy, or unable to reach the edge of the pond, the next area in which disease manifests is the inner tube. Therefore we must look at these two together.

As the outer tube, the skin is the foremost exposure to the outer world so amongst its functions is protection. Many of the forms acute illness takes arise from the function of the skin. The skin forms a barrier that seals in the organism and seals out the world. It has specialised cells to detect intrusion and repair injury promptly – see **Wounds** in Lesson 1 First Aid. It functions as a temperature regulator exchanging heat and protecting against cold to some degree – so it comes into *General* symptoms with fever, heat, cold, chill. As an organ of excretion it sweats – also a *General* symptom. It is well supplied with nerve endings to detect the presence of the outer world so it is often where **sensations** arise, especially expressed in pain. Acutes that reach the skin, reach the edge of the pond and usually resolution. In spots, pimples, rashes, and even ulcers, not to mention abscesses, disturbance is contained as *local* foci of *inflammation* and *suppuration*, and *ulceration*. Acute ailments often involve *general* metabolic symptoms such as fever, chill or malaise.

When acutes manifest in the inner tube, in the digestive system, some symptoms arise because of the nature of that tissue. In the respiratory system, we saw this as mucus membrane producing excess mucus discharge. While mucus production is marked in some remedies in the digestive system, in acute digestive complaints we see the action of the *system* rather than local disturbance – the best example is diarrhoea and vomit. *There may be a return to local disturbance of tissue in deeper disturbance such as gastric ulcers where structural change rather than dysfunction is the level of disturbance.* The reason for such activity at the system level is probably because a major function of the digestive system is excretion so, in the first instance, function is accelerated so excretion is increased as diarrhoea, with or without colic or vomit. This first action is common in children from slight causes such as overheating (*Belladonna*), or vexation (*Chamomilla*), or chill after overheating (*Dulcamara*). It parallels the defence response of *inflammation* in the psoric patient, but it is a deeper reaction of the Vital Force because it involves a *system.* In the instances given above, the clear *exciting causes* indicate a strong vitality despite involving the functioning of the system.

At the start of dysfunction, it is the rhythm that is changed, i.e. first, it is speeded up. This is easily seen in the digestive system where part of the function is rhythmic contraction which enables the movement of food and later faeces along the tube. Where there is deeper disturbance in the psoric patient we find the rhythm slows down, as in constipation – compare *Sulphur* and *Calcarea*. This may be the result of maintaining causes or be the nature of a more sluggish constitution. The Homoeopath will treat these two causes differently.

Where a system is disturbed, usually we look at the role of chronic [1] disease because system disturbance is a deeper adaptation of the Vital Force. The digestive system is an exception to this because it meets the external world through the food we take in. Thus, the digestive system needs protective measures like the skin. Its main protection that we see commonly in acute situations is vomit and diarrhoea by which it expels whatever is bothering it. It is this protective measure that becomes acutes in the digestive system.

The Maintaining Cause

The most common ailments in the digestive system caused by maintaining causes arise from bad eating habits or dietary indiscretion. Hence, *indigestion, heartburn, burping* and *flatulence* are all symptoms arising from the **maintaining cause** of eating too much, eating too rich food or food known to disagree, or eating too fast. Any mother will tell you the repercussions of chocolate cake, ice cream and jelly at a birthday party where the normal rules of one piece only, *'don't be greedy'*, are suspended for just a little while. Who has not tucked into a gourmet feast at Christmas or a special night out only to feel *nauseous with a heavy stomach*, even dull pain, relieved only by vomiting most of the contents of the stomach? Cream cakes, chocolate and alcohol are prime movers. When it comes to *flatulence,* we have all been warned about beans, brussels sprouts and onions. Some of us are more sensitive than others depending on our underlying predispositions. Acid foods may cause heartburn in most people in quantity but some are more sensitive because the cardiac sphincter of the stomach is weakened – often called a hiatus hernia by the doctor. In these types there is the distinctive modality of < lying down.

Note that there are two types of situations here. The first arises from the maintaining cause but the second including Individuality and Susceptibility has the exciting cause < acids. The Homoeopath will treat these differently. See below.

Other sore tummies from bad habit may arise indirectly because of constipation. More acutely, the gut may go into spasm to exert pressure on the food to move. In the longer term other symptoms arise, some with further consequences. A dull ache may occur as the wrong kind of food slows the gut. The slow action of the liver means it does not do its primary job of excreting toxins, products of catabolism, from the bloodstream. Such toxins lead to headaches and dullness of consciousness. Ultimately gout, acidic deposits in the joints, could be associated. Where the liver is congested constipation from poor diet may cause greasy spots in the teenager whose skin is already unbalanced by hormones – from the inner to the outer tube.

Later in life the menopausal woman or someone with years of little exercise may produce a similar congested picture that may lead to such a sluggish metabolism that gall stones may feature or even more degenerative diseases such as irritable bowel syndrome or even diverticular disease may appear. To the old Naturopaths constipation was the root of much lowered vitality and poor health. In this light it should be remembered that exercise that uses the big thigh muscles stimulates the flow of blood through the abdomen so exercise is as important for digestive health as a good diet.

Note that when the habits are changed the process may resolve itself if it has not gone too far. Where it has gone as far as diverticular disease other measures may be needed to preserve or promote functioning.

---

[1] *Chronic disease* has a special meaning in Homoeopathy. It is not determined by time as in orthodox medicine. In chronic disease the Homoeopath is identifying a fundamental change in the nature of the Vital Force – an adaptation or mutation – so functioning and presentation of symptoms is changed.

> **PRACTICE POINT**
>
> Always check diet and exercise regime in patients presenting with digestive disorders.

The Exciting Cause

These may fall into several categories. Since each constitution has its own **exciting cause** and weakness, we may find a complexity of causes such as chocolate, wine, cheese, etc giving rise to a range of ailments from *nausea, vomit, diarrhoea* to *travel sickness, colic, food poisoning, dysentery*. Some of these are symptoms whilst the same might also be an ailment in itself.

Children often produce a disorder in the digestive system on exposure to heat or cold, i.e. when others would produce a cold or flu. In other words, there may be an external trigger because of sensitivity or, more important to the Homoeopath, **susceptibility** may be an event waiting to happen because of the vitality and predispositions of the Vital Force. This last is the true homoeopathic acute so let us look further at susceptibility.

Kent speaks of Blackwater Fever that comes on *after exposure* to the evening *chill after the heat* of the day in Mid West USA in summer. He explains how *Dulcamara* fits this symptom picture well because of the symptoms of *watery diarrhoea* and the **exciting cause** < *chill after overheating*. This is the reaction of a rheumatoid remedy [2] of which *Dulcamara* is a good example. When generally disturbed it throws out the disturbance depending on its vitality. In a less vital patient the manifestation may be paralysis as in rheumatism. *Chamomilla* is an example of a child's remedy where the diarrhoea is produced due to susceptibility at the system level – we talk of **affinity** in the digestive system. In the case of *Chamomilla* green, sour-smelling diarrhoea is produced *on teething* or as a result of *vexation*, being thwarted. Both remedies produce diarrhoea characteristically but the **exciting causes** are very different. In *Dulcamara*, there is a rheumatic tendency that is susceptible to cold. In *Chamomilla* teething is a metabolic change whilst vexation is emotional. In *Chamomilla* there is sensitivity of the nervous system.

The acute is produced according to the predisposition of the Vital Force, the characteristic pattern of manifestation, the where and how of symptoms, that includes the **susceptibility,** that to which it resonates, which then determines the exciting cause to which the patient will react.

The acute may have nothing to do with habit in the digestive system. Travel sickness is a good example here. Tiredness, as a maintaining cause, may predispose to travel sickness. Eating too many sweets, as a maintaining cause, may make the child prone on that occasion but there may be an underlying constitution that makes some more prone than others. Thus, some patients have known triggers, **exciting causes,** and an individual symptom picture with its own Strange, Rare and Peculiars, characteristic symptoms and modalities. Disorientation, stress to the system and the autonomic nervous system seem to have much to do with travel sickness. This can be seen clearly in remedies useful for travel sickness, such as *Ignatia* and *Ipecacuanha* which have a strong effect on the autonomic nervous system but produce their own distinct symptom pictures – see below. **Individuality** is often found in the **modalities** of some of the travel sickness remedies – < tobacco, > closing the eyes, > open air – that also show the effect of the autonomic nervous system.

Food poisoning is an acute with an external cause. Some people are more susceptible than others but there is a degree to which we will all react. Whilst the orthodox practitioner will regard food poisoning as falling into different categories depending on whether the bacterium produces the toxins immediately or later, the Homoeopath selects a remedy according to the uniqueness of the symptom picture, i.e. the **Individuality**. The Homoeopath has remedies such as *Arsenicum* that produce an immediate and violent response of vomiting and diarrhoea, or remedies like *Nux vomica* whose action is spasm, including projectile vomiting.

---

[2] Rheumatism is a deeper disturbance manifesting in the middle tube. The earlier stages of the chronic disease are therefore often found in the inner tube, or even outer tube if we look at the many skin problems of *Rhus toxicodendron*.

The **essence** of *Arsenicum* is extreme sensitivity to anything out of order. The essence of *Nux vomica* is very similar – out of harmony. In seeking for further **Individuality,** the Homoeopath will find *Nux vomica* has the keynote symptom *if only I could be sick.* Further, *Nux vomica* is < *heat* whereas *Arsenicum* is *generally > heat* and has *burning pains > heat.* Vithoulkas criteria of **Accuracy** and **Precision** are essential to a good homoeopathic prescription based in **Individuality** and **Susceptibility**.

This method of working is irrespective of germ theory. The Homoeopath simply matches the symptom picture (thereby dismissing millions of pounds of research and animal sacrifice). This is equally the procedure with acute disease such as dysentery and cholera, much more extreme forms of food poisoning caused by exposure of the digestive system to virulent alien organisms, usually when their vitality is already under stress. Following Bechamp the Homoeopath sees germs as scavengers that can only thrive where the soil is right for them, i.e. where there is disorder. It is important to remember that the gut has colonies of friendly organisms that promote its function of digesting foodstuffs. Healthy gut organisms such as lactophiliac bacteria need an alkaline environment. E Coli is just one of the bacteria that grow in more acid environments – such as those produced by sugar and salt imbibing. This leads us back to the maintaining cause and good habits although some constitutions by the nature of their chronic case are predisposed or more prone than others – back to the fact that the Homoeopath treats the Individual, always.

Potency

When the cause is an exciting cause, the Homoeopath may reach for a 6 - 30th potency to correct the disturbance of the Vital Force. This may depend on the sensitivity of the patient, the severity of the symptom picture and whether there are any blocks to the action of the Vital Force. Someone with a more reactive Vital Force like a child may need only a 6th potency but where **susceptibility** is greater a higher potency may be needed – this would then be indicated by a more severe reaction or severity of the symptom picture. The Homoeopath always looks at the Total Symptom Picture and it is this action that identifies blocks to cure. An example of a block might be constitutional sluggishness with constipation – then the Homoeopath may prefer to start the treatment more slowly with the 6th potency to avoid severe aggravation as the drain is cleared! This may be an occasion to repeat the dose as needed, i.e. each evening until a more regular pattern is established. Where there is much dehydration and tenemus, as in the diarrhoea of the visitor to very hot countries, it may be better to start with a 200th potency because the symptoms are affecting the patient on the *General* level. Such a severe case may need help to rehydrate.

The potency used is chosen in relation to the speed of action of the Vital Force which is indicated by the severity of the symptom picture and the speed with which it appears. Severity is directly related to discomfort (!) and the type of symptom presented. Movement from the local (*particular*) symptom to the *General* is a sure sign of a deepening crisis, as is movement of symptoms from *sensation* to *dysfunction* type when the activity is in a *system.* Whilst we may raise the potency from particular to general, we will lower it from sensation to dysfunction. We must learn to understand what the symptoms are telling us.

The difficulty for the beginner is when to repeat the dose. The golden rule in Homoeopathy is of course *never to repeat the dose.* It is best to match the energy of the Vital Force to the energy of the remedy and choose an appropriate potency. When I started to practise I did not understand Homoeopathy and used Split Doses (2 pills, one before bed and the other next morning) and Collective Single Doses (a pill at three hourly intervals for 3 doses). I was amazed when I learned to read the symptoms and saw how powerful a single pill was. At the start it is better to go higher than needed, although a 30th potency was the highest Hahnemann used, so you can clearly see the change in the symptom picture and follow Hering's Laws of Cure. The patient may be overly aggravated but your future patients will be much better off as a result of your confidence! But remember we are talking of acute cases here. Where a chronic case is using the digestive system as a drain, it is not advisable to increase the speed of excretion as there may be much much more to come.

So when do we repeat the dose?

Hopefully, if the potency was well chosen, there is no need to repeat the dose. In a digestive complaint where vomit or diarrhoea is a symptom, there may be another evacuation after the remedy, then the body will enter a rest phase in which it can recuperate. All is well.

However, we may find that we have only decreased the intensity, or frequency. This is not yet cure. We can say the process of cure has started if there is change in the type of symptom, i.e. if the *General* symptoms are lessened, even if the *particulars* are worse. The best homoeopathic prescription is to **wait** but how long do you wait with vomit or diarrhoea? An hour if it is not too severe? Has the rest period started? What is the difference between exhaustion and rest? One is a dullness and lack of energy. **Check** if the symptom picture agrees with that of the remedy you have used. Any change in the kind of symptoms at this point must be viewed with suspicion. One of Vithoulkas' criteria is the rise in energy level. If this is present there is no problem we must wait. All is well.

If there is no significant change except in frequency and intensity, and even that is not very impressive, then think of a higher potency – this is especially so if only a 6th potency was used.

Where the situation was severe and the change is now from *General* to more severe *particular*, i.e. the fever has abated but the diarrhoea may be worse you might repeat a 30th potency (although it is better to **plus** this) or give a higher potency. Traditionally the higher potency to the 30th would have been the 200th. Today's people are more chronically diseased with poor vitality so this may be an enormous leap. Plussing [3] is an ideal solution here. Otherwise, I keep acute remedies in intermediate potencies such as the 60th and the 100th.

Always be guided by the change in symptoms.

Where there is really no change and you have waited long enough, you have probably given the wrong remedy although it may be too low a potency.

Where the maintaining cause is the problem it may be better to use repeat doses of the 6th potency **as needed** whilst the change of habit gets to the root of the problem, i.e. as the body copes with the excess volume of food or alcohol after a celebration. Here there is a question as to the meaning of 'when needed'.

PRACTICE POINT

It is easier to read a change in the symptom picture, or to follow the progress of change, if you have selected clear *indicating symptoms*, e.g. vomit and diarrhoea but also sweat, chill, fever or even better symptoms of Individuality like *if only I could be sick*.

Questions to ask before selecting a potency

- How sensitive is the patient?
- How fast is the Vital Force working?
- At what level are the symptom produced?
- If severe, what are the criteria for severity?

---

[3] Put a pill of whatever potency you have previously used into some water, a teaspoonful is enough, then vigorously shake this before giving it to the patient.

Questions to ask before changing a potency

- What has changed? Intensity? Frequency? Type of symptom? Energy level?
- If all four, **wait.**
- If only Intensity and Frequency, consider plussing.
- If Generals better and particulars worse, either wait or increase potency.

Questions to ask before changing the remedy

- Is there really no change in the symptoms?
- If new symptoms, where are they coming from? The remedy? A deeper constitutional disturbance?
- What is happening to the general symptoms, the energy levels, the indicating symptoms?

> **EXERCISE**
>
> There can be no substitute here for observation. Watch the changing pattern of symptoms in acute illness of self and family.
>
> Are you able to find symptoms of Individuality or Susceptibility?
>
> Can you isolate *Indicating symptoms*?
>
> What happens to these after the remedy is given?
>
> Does the patient's energy change?
>
> How do you measure this?

ANATOMY AND PHYSIOLOGY

The digestive system is a tube that stretches from the mouth to the anus. It takes in solid and liquid physical matter at one end, extracts nutrients from this and expels the debris at the other end. It secretes digestive enzymes to dissolve selectively nutrients before absorbing them into the 'interior'. Its function in handling alien materials brings the outside world within the system. It is a primary interface with the external world. The symptoms of vomit and diarrhoea are violent excretory motions that rapidly expel the foreign material and the debris that could be potentially damaging. Thus as well as symptoms these are defence mechanisms.

The liver is one of its specialised organs, which extracts the products of catabolism and secretes them into the gut for excretion from the system. The liver also acts as a transformer station processing the energy extracted from food into a form more readily available to the body. The glucose produced by the digestive enzymes from carbohydrates is stored in the liver as glycogen to be converted and released when needed as glucose into the bloodstream.

The pancreas on the left side opposite the liver creates enzymes to digest protein and carbohydrates.

The stomach is a swollen part of the tube that produces its own enzymes. It is a bag that acts as a first receiving station for the food after the mouth. Its churning action mixes the food finely with the enzymes. The largest section of the tube, the small intestine, absorbs nutrients prepared specially for absorption. The large intestine is swollen like the stomach. Food lies there longer than in the small intestine so that fluid can be reabsorbed and recycled.

Movement along the whole of the tube is by peristalsis. Like a worm, circular muscles contract in a wave-like pattern pushing food along the gut. When this peristaltic movement increases, the speed of food passage increases causing diarrhoea at one end. If violent and reversed at the start of the tube, it produces vomiting. Where extremely severe, contraction reverses peristalsis producing cramps or even faecal vomiting, as in *Nux vomica*.

> **EXERCISE**
>
> Study the Anatomy and Physiology in more detail in a relevant textbook.
>
> Draw a diagram to show you know the component parts and how they fit together.
>
> Study the enzymes of digestion. Where are they found in the gut and what do they digest?

Remedies of Travel Sickness

Ipecacuanha is a remedy of collapsed, over-relaxed constitutions. It easily produces *vomit with all complaints*, e.g. even with cough, because its **affinity** is for the autonomic nervous system. The action of the ANS through the pneumo-gastric nerve is to create relaxation that results in copious flow, i.e. *copious mucus* with the vomit. The role of the autonomic nervous system means there is *no relief* after the contents are expelled. The patient continues to feel nauseous and vomits. In accompanying symptoms, the stomach may be so relaxed it feels as if it is *hanging down*. In the child disturbance may easily go on to produce diarrhoea that is *green and slimy*. The patient is *aggravated from the slightest motion*. << stooping. > fresh air.

Ignatia is weakened by emotional distress. It is a spasmodic remedy that particularly affects the diaphragm via the vagus nerve so *sighing* is a feature. It is very sensitive to *tobacco* which is a major irritant of smooth muscle of which the gut is largely composed. Thus the nausea and vomit is violent but > *fresh air*. The nervous involvement here means you may see them *tremble and shake*, i.e. the remedy acts more *generally*. Causation is more often the nervous system than digestive, although digestion is affected by nervous disorder.

Nux vomica may have travel sickness because they have eaten too much or too rich food, i.e. **maintaining cause**. They are *worse from the heat* within a vehicle – digestion creates much heat already. This is also a remedy of the nervous system but the symptom is *over stimulation*. Often the nervous system is *exhausted* so the travel sickness may be > *closing the eyes*. Over stimulation may be seen in the keynote, reversed *peristalsis*, so you will hear them retch and say '*If only I could be sick*'. Once they vomit, they are usually much better but the **essence** of *Nux vomica* is *out of harmony*. Nothing is right.

Cocculus has a *profuse flow of saliva* and is *< for the smell of food* because this causes the gastric juices to flow. The ANS is responsible for relaxation and greater *flow* but here the Central Nervous System is involved so they *lose co-ordination and feel most unsteady, as if at sea*. Indeed the *nausea seems to rise up to the head* as the sensory nerves are disrupted. Nervous involvement is seen in the **modalities**. *< loss of sleep,* noise or touch.

Remedies of Food Poisoning

Arsenicum   is a very sensitive remedy with a clear idea of what is in the right place. They are *fastidious* and extremely well-organised in order to cope with their anxiety, **essence,** so their response to food poisoning is immediate and severe. Sudden nausea and *prostration* plus heat in the stomach may proceed the vomiting. After rest, they may be fine. If it goes further they will produce *foul-smelling diarrhoea* that is *watery*. The more severe the attack the worse the smell so it can *smell like decaying rotten meat* and the more watery the diarrhoea the more *excoriating,* burning the anus. They are extremely *chilly, losing vital* heat so you will find them wrapped in blankets. This remedy shows **individuality** of symptoms related to the **essence,** tension compensating for disintegration so the 'attack' of food poisoning achieves an effect that is out of proportion.

Nux vomica   has heat in the abdomen, nausea and colic. Unlike *Arsenicum,* they are < *heat*. '*If only I could be sick or pass a stool*' is the dominant symptom. There may be a headache develop on the *vertex as of a weight pressing down*. At other times, *anger* is the **exciting cause.** They are noted for their scowl contorting their face. We call it sour-faced. The gut reacts to food poisoning in a similar way as if drawn together by a lemon. The gut is over-contracted so nothing can pass. They will even say they felt 'poisoned'. Here again, you see how the **essence** creates **individuality**.

> **EXERCISE**
>
> It is such a skill to pick out the symptoms of a case so, just to drive home the values, use coloured pencils to identify or highlight the symptoms above of:
>
> Exciting Cause
> Location
> Sensation
> Modality

Remedies of Colic

Colic is a common acute of the digestive system. It may arise from a **maintaining cause** as greater contraction resulting from over-rich food or it may arise from an **exciting cause** expressing **spasm** as the inflammatory level of disease process. If we use a homoeopathic remedy the cause may be irrelevant except the exciting cause is part of the symptom picture, and symptoms arising from a maintaining cause may be speeded up as to their resolution but will not be removed until the cause itself is removed and/or its effects healed.

Belladonna   has violent, *shooting, stitching pains with heat* in the abdomen. In the head, these may become pulsations. The patient groans constantly. Their symptoms are *worse eating* although they are mentally better eating. The tongue is *red with white papillae* showing disturbance in the system. In gastralgia *the pains shoot up the spine*. There is *pressure* as if the contents of the abdomen would come out of the stomach, i.e. a **sensation** of bursting. The colic may proceed the diarrhoea *after a cold*. The diarrhoea may then be *slimy and bloody,* > *lying on the abdomen*.

Note, the **exciting cause** here is < after cold, whilst the **modality** is < eating. *Belladonna* may also produce this inflammatory condition after heat or sunstroke. This may present in the digestive system.

Chamomilla occurs frequently in *teething* babies or in children who are < *after anger*. The mental syndrome should dominate so you will notice the *capriciousness* before the *green sour smelling diarrhoea* appears. Indeed, the diarrhoea appears after the temper tantrum. Their only relief is *being carried* around; in digestive upset they will *press the abdomen into your shoulder, > pressure*. Capriciousness corresponds to the **essence** of over-sensitivity or easily offended, the keynote is < vexation.

Colocynth is often recommended for children with colic. If it is the indicated remedy they twist and turn restlessly and bend double, especially *after eating and drinking*, **modality.** The pains are *better for pressure in the abdomen* so you will find them *lying on their abdomen*. Indeed, they can be so distressed you will find them pressing the corners of the table into the abdomen. Like *Chamomilla* the condition may be brought on *after anger*, **exciting cause**. Pain will centre on the navel and come in *spasms every 5-10 minutes, > passing flatus*. Were they able to describe the pain they might say it was like *two stones grinding* or as if a *knife were twisted in their gut*. There is vomit and diarrhoea with the colic. This remedy has an **affinity** for the nervous system so it comes as no surprise to see so many symptoms of **sensation.**

Ipecacuanha has a *cutting pain around the umbilical region*. There is *much flatulence* and *nausea*. Saliva will be copious. If there is vomit it will have much mucus in its content. Even when very ill, the tongue is clean showing the **affinity** is of the autonomic nervous system rather than digestive system. Their appetite is affected so they *desire what are called 'dainties'* in the *Materia Medica* books. This is similar to *Ignatia* that has a *contrary appetite* desiring things like tomato sauce you would expect to make them worse. The *Ipecacuanha* patient tends to be a negative type if you listen to the content of their gossip.

The **essence** of this remedy would include relaxation, letting go, letting things go to the dogs even, hence the mucus in the vomit as the stomach releases gastric juices, having let go of the *natural appetite they grasp or crave the unnatural, the gossip can then also be seen as a letting go*. The **exciting cause** is thus factors that contribute to this relaxation, i.e. stress, usually by further pressurising the organism as is easily seen in travel sickness. There may not be a clear exciting cause but look how the **individuality** of the symptoms follows that of an acute produced by an **exciting cause.**

Magnesium phosphoricum is a major homeopathic anti-spasmodic, though think also of *Belladonna* and *Nux vomica* especially in where sphincters go into spasm. The difference with *Magnesium phosphoricum* is that the pains *suddenly come and go, like lightning*, **sensation**, and are > *heat and pressure*, **modality,** so the patient *holds the abdomen* or bends double. The pain may be as if there were a *band around the body*. There is *belching with the colic*. And there is a *great dread of uncovering or of getting the part cold*. The **exciting cause** is described as *standing in cold water* (*Pulsatilla* and *Rhus toxicodendron* are worse getting the feet wet). The *headache starts at the back* and *extends over the head* to end in a red face (as in *Pulsatilla* and different from *Nux vomica* where the headache is on the vertex (**location**).

Nux vomica is one of the major remedies of the intestines because of its spasmodic action on peristalsis. The keynote is 'If only I could be ...' – usually it is 'sick'. This remedy can cause such *violent colic* it produces faecal vomiting or even intersuccussion where the intestine loops into itself. Pain is < heat. Usually the spasm arises out of tension or even anger. This patient's nerves are so sensitive they are frequently *irritable*. Irritable in the digestive system is **spasm**. The sense organs are *oversensitive* so **modalities** include < *noise* and < *light*. Tobacco is often an **exciting cause. Maintaining causes** include coffee, alcohol and *stimulating foods*.

Note: the face often shows *Nux vomica* in its scowl, or ' the sour face'.

Remedies of Dysentery

Dysentery is much more severe than diarrhoea. It involves exposure to external factors. These attack those resonant or lacking in vitality, e.g. children and old people are especially vulnerable. With both these groups, there is the added danger of fluid loss that may leach electrolytes giving the added problems of cramps.

It is important to remember that Homoeopathy treats the individual so there are as many remedies of dysentery as there are people. Even where there is a known labelled disease and cause, as Homoeopaths we look for the factors that engage the Vital Force, those to which it is resonant, i.e. we build up the individual symptom picture. Symptoms of **Individuality** and **Susceptibility** will enable us to differentiate accurately remedies. These include **exciting causes, modalities** and **sensations.**

The way in which an individual reacts to any factor, such as dirty water or food poisoning, will depend on his/her underlying predisposition. Hence, some are more prone to dysentery than others because there is an **affinity for** the digestive system – these types may be better treated constitutionally, i.e. as prevention. When working out the potential remedies for those going abroad it is necessary to look at the constitutional weaknesses to determine the related acute remedies.

Because dysentery is more violent, the Homoeopath will use the higher potencies, 200th or 1M. Where the single dose is used, the patient will be expected to go back to the toilet once more then fall into a deep and restful state.

Arsenicum Whilst the smell will drive you from the sick room, the most pronounced effect will be on the patient's Mental and Emotional state. Diarrhoea quickly *prostrates* and anxiety arises. Anxiety and *fear of cholera* becomes great *restlessness* then *prostration out of all proportion*. They *dread death* and would rather kill themselves than suffer so they believe *they are incurable* and it is pointless to take the medicine. There is a *cold sweat on a pale face*. The *burning pains* are so fierce they describe them as like *coals of fire*. There is *watery offensive diarrhoea* that *smells like rotten meat* and *burns and corrodes the anus* as it passes. The diarrhoea is *worse for eating or drinking* yet they have a *great thirst for cold water* that is taken in little sips, *little and often*. Although *hot, they are better for heat* but want the *head cool*. They are << *cold food and drink*.
Note that in comparing this with the *Arsenicum* mentioned above, the symptoms are more severe and there are stronger Mental and Emotional symptoms. Emphasis is very important in homoeopathic prescriptions.

Mercurius has *bloody, offensive stools*. The *mouth feels slimy*. There is a *metallic taste*. There is often *mucus in the stool*. They have *tenesmus (*straining*) even with diarrhoea*. It is as if they are unable to evacuate fully the bowel. They have a *never-get-done feeling* (*Nux vomica* has a feeling as if there is still something in the rectum.) *Straining goes on even after the stool* so they can even expel the rectum. There is *great burning* in the anus after the stool. They are worse at night and on any motion. Often the *bladder is also involved with slimy, bloody urine*. The may become faint and *chilly* afterwards. This is a remedy of the syphilitic miasm. Note the burning and bloodiness and the intensity of the destruction.

> **EXERCISE**
>
> Read over *Arsenicum* and *Mercurius* above to highlight the following:
>
> Individuality
> Susceptibility
> Affinity
> Sensation
> Modality
> Exciting Cause

> **EXERCISE**
>
> There is a great deal of information above that could be more easily accessed in a table. Following the pattern in Lesson 4, list the Exciting Causes alphabetically with associated remedies. Create an alphabetical list of sensations with associated remedies. They were clever and diligent people who created repertories! Now list the modalities with their remedies.

Remedies

Arsenicum album

This is a remedy for the active type of patient. Whilst others may have ideas, the *Arsenicum* patient makes it happen. They are driven by an underlying insecurity so organising their world is making it safe. This is the control freak but do not forget they really are adept at getting things done. They are *fastidious* and *restless,* always on the go. They appear to have volumes of energy but you can imagine the strain on the integrity of the organism created by so much tension.

Any *Arsenicum* illness is characterised by the speed of onset accompanied by *great prostration, out of all proportion.* There may be a sudden shock to their organisation, such as a new director (they are usually the managers of industry, if not the director). Any loss of face, an attack on their self esteem, will assault the integrity of the organism so they sink fast. The same volume of energy that created the organisation is now turned in to create the illness.

At the first level of acute, the more healthy type may produce profuse watery discharge from the nose especially if the weather is cold. The *Arsenicum* patient is one of the four chilliest remedies in the whole *Materia Medica.* Think of that a little. In Homoeopathy, we call chilliness *lack of vital heat.* This wording may help you see why chilliness is such an attack on the integrity of the whole. Chilliness accompanies all *Arsenicum* symptoms and cold is both an exciting cause and a modality.

Another characteristic of *Arsenicum* is right-sidedness. So in the profuse nasal discharge above we have the individuality of running only from the right nostril. Another characteristic is corrosiveness of discharges so above the skin under the right nostril quickly becomes raw, a terrible affliction for one who is so fastidious.

Another common acute of *Arsenicum* is diarrhoea. In keeping with the essential nature of the remedy, there is over-action so the digestive system is speeded up. The individuality is an excoriating watery stool that burns causing rawness of the anus. Further individuality is the smell that resembles *rotten meat or carcasses.* And, of course, the patient is very chilly and very prostrate, suddenly. *Arsenicum* is a common remedy of food poisoning because essentially it is very sensitive to anything out of order. The old textbooks tell us they are especially sensitive to rotten meat or fish. Think of the type of bacteria that cause such poisoning. The *Arsenicum* patient is so sensitive that the reaction will set in rapidly, and even after they have eaten the same food as others.

Digestive symptoms feature strongly in the constitutional case. If you think of it, they are sensitive to any influence from the outside world and the digestive system is a major point of entry of the outside world in the shape of food. The *Arsenicum* patient *cannot stand the sight or smell of food.* It brings on nausea. They may eat little and often or one big meal per day. Eating little and often is characteristic of the patient with indigestion or ulcers and the *Arsenicum* patient is prone to both of these. Indigestion takes the form of *burning pains.* The individuality of these is *burning pains > heat.*

Were we to look deeper into the constitutional picture, we would see the effects of the stress continual organisation causes. When the integrity of the whole is affected in this very individual person, it is the heart and circulation that are weakened so this patient is prone to *hypertension* (high blood pressure), to gastric ulcers, and heart problems arising from arterial sclerosis – adrenaline releases fat from storage and without actual physical activity this is laid down between the walls of the arteries to create inflexibility. Rheumatism and peripheral oedema may be a protective earlier stage, or a later complication. The acute illness will most probably then occur in the respiratory system, i.e. a deeper system than digestive. *Arsenicum* is one of the remedies of pneumonia or fluid problems in the lungs of aged persons.

Ipecacuanha

This is an interesting remedy with a strong effect on the pneumo-gastric nerve. Whilst it may produce spasm in its first action, very like *Ignatia*, its main characteristic is collapse or *laxity*. Almost all conditions are accompanied by *nausea*. Thus the main acutes are digestive.

Where the nervous system is disturbed, as in the vibrations of travel, nausea rises. Unfortunately, they will vomit and *vomit without relief* because the disturbance only manifests in the digestive system – it is the nervous system that is really disturbed. The Autonomic Nervous System controls the functioning of the digestive system, the rhythm of peristalsis and the degree of secretion. Hence, the relaxed tissue secretes mucus so the vomit may contain *tenacious, white, glairy mucus*. When the situation is severe, the laxity increases so there is a sensation *as if the stomach hung down*. Bouts of vomit are followed by exhaustion so they become *sleepy after vomiting*. This will give you an idea as to how much energy is expended, indeed as to how violent the attacks can be.

The digestive system is easily distressed by heavy fatty food such as *pork and pastries* – as in *Pulsatilla*. Vomit is the first answer to such insult – spit it back out again, not to take in the poisoning. Constitutionally since they have a desire for delicacies, they frequently overindulge leading to *flatulence* and *cutting colic around the umbilical region,* like *Pulsatilla* and *Chamomilla*. As in *Chamomilla*, the stool may be green. It is frequently full of slimy mucus as in *Mercurius*. The individuality that distinguishes *Ipecacuanha* in these cases is the *clean tongue* because disturbance is basically of the nerves. Where the tongue is coated, it is only slight because the remedy is so reactive it keeps the digestive system healthily reactive and therefore clear.

I passed over the spasm above. The mode with which the digestive system responds is through spasm that produces the diarrhoea or vomit but in deeper disturbance of the constitution it occurs in deeper more important systems. The digestive system is the first defence because it is excretory, but cold weather may bring the cough, or even *croup*. Of course cough is spasm, a natural defence to expel anything from the respiratory system to protect the vital organ of the lungs. The young child will become *rigid* or even *blue with spasm*. More usually, the spasm is so intense it sets off the gastric side of the pneumo-gastric nerve so they *choke and gag till they vomit*, as in *Drosera*. The tendency to suffocate in the spasm makes *Ipecacuanha* one of the main acute remedies of asthma when there is mucus present.

Its other important use in the First Aid box is for haemorrhage. *Small wounds bleed profusely* because the tissue is so lax. The blood is bright red as opposed to *Carbo vegetalis* where lax tissue leads to small wounds bleeding profuse dark venous blood. *Carbo vegetalis* is a remedy of broken down constitutions whereas in *Ipecacuanha* lax tissue is activated by the Autonomic Nervous System. *Ipecacuanha* can be a remedy of arterial bleeding which spurts spasmodically as the artery contracts – every remedy has its opposite symptom! It can be indicated after childbirth for uterine haemorrhage where the muscle is tired and over-relaxed. Individuality is indicated by *nausea* and *heavy breathing*. Much breathing is of course controlled by the pneumo-gastric nerve. This symptom can be looked at in relation to the sighing of the *Ignatia* patient.

Constitutionally, the *Ipecacuanha* patient is one of Jane Austen's young ladies – nervous, sensitive and over-reactive. Remedies of the Autonomic Nervous System are anxious and on the alert. For what?

Look how she is put out of harmony and collapses. It is not the faint of *Ignatia*. Her body takes control and she produces *nausea* that is very debilitating so she is exhausted after it. Diarrhoea and other spasm is the body taking over as it separates or contains the emotional trauma. Thus, she is alienated from herself. Her view of life is negative. It attacks. She is helpless. So she is a disagreeable type. Some would point her out as the negative neighbour who has nothing but bad to say of others. In such a state she allows life to sit on her, having no get up and go to rise to a challenge. Thus she will wear you down leaving you feeling as helpless as her.

Ignatia

This is another of Jane Austen's young ladies. She is inclined to faint on hearing bad news or, love-lorn, she will *not be able to eat or sleep from thinking* of him. As a remedy of the vagus nerve it affects the diaphragm – think of the corsets worse by Victorian ladies!

In the First Aid box, Ignatia is a remedy of emotional shock. It is as if they draw in their breath but cannot come back into the world. Breathe you want to say but they are *benumbed*. They will keep reliving the moment of impact as if they seized up at that point. Their talk and dreams are full of the image of the shock. In particular the shock concerns the loss of a loved one, through *grief* or *disappointed love*. They are prone to disappointment in love because they most often choose *inappropriate objects for their attention*. They are idealists or romantics. As idealists they follow causes. On one level they have great energy but they are also prone to *hysteria*, going over the top. I often recognise them because they are scattered all over the room and it takes me time to collect them together to find out what they want! The separation from reality increases in degree. From the moping of the teenager's first love, it may become the cold stony *silent grief* that cannot express itself, or even the *inappropriate laughter* displayed by a patient who found her mum hanged. The feelings are so intense they are denied or even displaced. At first there is an intensity that holds on then it is pushed away. This parallels the physical realm that has spasm in the first action then relaxation.

Spasm gives rise to such symptoms as the *globus hystericum*, the lump in the throat. The remedy is useful for trips to the dentist when the lump in the throat causes them to swallow continually and so choke. The spasm in the diaphragm produces *sighing* in emotional situations, or even hiccoughs. They may even *yawn spasmodically*. When the sensitivity expresses in digestive conditions, it produces vomit which is a spasm. Their sensitivity has the modality of worse tobacco hence travel sickness arises in a carriage full of *tobacco smoke* – except, they are so sensitive, they can smell the slightest whiff of tobacco. Or, was it tobacco? Because *thinking makes it so*, they can be nauseous from thinking someone is smoking.

They are contradictory types, fickle in nature. Even their symptoms are *contrary*. Although nauseous, they will eat food that would make you and me worse. They have a liking for tomato sauce! The remedy contains more strychnine than *Nux vomica* but here the action affects the nervous system more strongly, especially the vagus nerve, so causing nausea or fainting. They *tremble with emotions*.

The headache is like a nail driven into the temple. The have *pains in small spots*. Once again that makes me think of Jane Austen young ladies, or the one with the spotty dress. They have a sense of what is right. As an acute remedy to *Natrum muriaticum*, they are very honest and forthright, even if naively so. With their refined nervous system, this should give a clue to their exciting causes as events that do not fit into their high ideals, or perfect world.

Colocynth

This is another remedy whose primary action is in the nervous system producing spasm. I have put it in here because I come across it frequently abused because used routinely and in high potency (30C) for colic in young babies!

The primary location of the acute is in the digestive system where it produces *colicky pains around the navel* as if the guts were *ground between two stones*. The spasms come *5-10 minutes apart* relieved only by *bending double*, or by *something pressed hard into the abdomen* (as in *Chamomilla*). The pain is so severe the patient is extremely irritable and does not want attention. (Compare with *Chamomilla* who *sends the 'nurse' from the room*, or *Bryonia* who is *very touchy when questioned*.) They withdraw into themselves eventually because any movement further stimulates the nerves. Eating or drinking the least amount aggravates. We need to differentiate between this remedy and *Lycopodium* where the pattern is 'eats in small amounts because easily filled' – in fact, the *Colocynth* patient becomes bloated as each mouthful quickly turns into wind.

Now you will see part of the problem. We need to split hairs to get the precise meaning of the symptom. When we are dealing with a baby who cannot speak to us, how do we get an accurate rendering of the symptom? This is when the modalities and the exciting cause can help. We can observe when the condition is better or worse. If we observe the point of change, we might identify the exciting cause. In the case of *Colocynth*, the exciting cause is *Anger*. An offence is internalised giving rise to *indignation* (see also *Staphisagria*). You can feel the body draw up into a tight spasm. It may be released as anger but the reaction may be so intense it is somatised as spasm in the digestive system. Now, if this is to be a remedy of colic in babies, ask yourself what they could possibly experience that could cause such violence. Bad food? A residue in Mum's milk (possibly of *her* emotions)? What kind of sensitivity would predispose them to this reaction? When older the child *will throw things* as in *Nux vomica* and *Chamomilla*. Note the strong centrifugal tendency to expel disturbance. But the agitation is deep and they are sleepless *after anger*. They cannot let go, as in *Staphisagria*. There is a persistent *bitter taste in their mouth*.

The spasm affects muscles so when the disease process deepens, the limbs are affected. *The limbs are drawn up* in colic. In rheumatism, which is *right sided*, there is a distinct sensation *as if the part were shortened. Cutting pains move down* the limbs. A specific location for rheumatism is the psoas muscle at the hip. Sciatic pains shoot down to the feet. They find relief *lying on painful parts* to stop the spasm. Spasms come in bouts 5 – 10 minutes apart here too.

This is one of the remedies (*Nux vomica* and *Chamomilla*) that find *relief in coffee* that can relax nerves, or cause greater tension after prolonged use. *Colocynth* has the *twitching muscles* of the heavy coffee drinker.

SHORT REPERTORY OF DIGESTIVE SYMPTOMS

Nausea	with abdominal pain	*arn*, **ars**, coloc, nux v, **sep**
	> open air	phos, *puls*
	After anxiety	nux v
	During backache	coloc
	After beer	bry, lach, nux v
	With chilliness	*lach, puls*
	On closing the eyes	*lach*
	After cold drinks	*ars*, lach, *nat m*, puls, *rhus t*
	> after cold drinks	*puls*
	< after eating	arn, ars, *bry*, coloc, hep, ign, *lach*, merc, *nat m*, **nux v**, **puls**, *rhus t, ruta*, **sep**, sil
	> eating	acon, bry, **sep**
	on looking at food	sil
	On the smell of food	*ars, sep*
	From rich food	**puls**, sep
	During headache	acon, arn, *ars, bry*, cimic, *coloc*, gels, hep, ign, *lach*, merc, nat m, nux v, *puls*, rhus t, ruta, *sep*, sil
	< after ice cream	*ars*, **puls**
	during labour	**puls**

	< on lying down	ars, puls, rhus t
	> lying down	arn, sep, sil
	< before menses	*nat m*, nux v, *puls,* sep
	< during menses	arn, ars, bell, *bry,* gels, nat m, nux v, *puls,* sep
	from suppressed menses (e.g. after contraceptive pill)	ars, nat m, *nux v,* **puls,** rhus t
	< on motion	*arn, bry,* hep, sep
	< on motion of the eyes	puls, sep
	from odours	sep
	during pain	ars, nat m, sep,
	during perspiration	merc, nux v, *sep*
	on raising the head from the pillow	*ars, bry*
	while reading	arn, sep
	with salivation	*nux v*, puls
	in seasickness	nat m, nux v, *sep*
	suddenly whilst eating	ruta
	< thinking of it	lach, sep
	after vaccination	**sil**
	whilst walking	acon, bell, bry, led, *sep,* sil
	< warm drinks	*lach,* **puls**
	< in a warm room	*puls,* sep
	when yawning	arn, nat m
Vomit	after anger	**coloc, nux v**
	on coughing	*arn, ars,* **bry,** gels, **hep,** *lach,* merc, *nat m nux v puls,* rhus t, *sep, sil,*
	during diarrhoea	**ars,** coloc, lach, merc, *puls,* sep
	after cold water	arn, ars, *bry,* gels, nux v, *sil*
	immediately after drinking	**ars, bry,** *nux v,*sep
	suddenly while eating	*ars,* puls, rhus t, sep, sil
	during headache	arn, ars, *bell,* bry, coloc, *gels, lach,* nat m, *nux v,* **puls,** sep, sil
	during heat	acon, *ars,* bell, *bry,* hep, ign, lach, **nat m,** nux v, puls
	before menstruation	gels, *nux v, puls*
	after drinking milk	*ars,* bell, lach, merc, *sep,* **sil**
	< on motion	**ars, bry,** *lach,* nux v
	painful	arn, *ars,* nat m
	during pregnancy	acon, *ars, bry, lach, nat m,* **nux v,** *puls,* **sep,** *sil*
	after rich food	*puls*
	during vertigo	*ars,* cimic, *lach,* merc, *nux v, puls,* sep
	of bile	*acon,* **ars,** *bell,* **bry,** *coloc,* hep, *ign, lach,* **merc,** *nat m,* **nux v, puls,** rhus t, **sep,** sil
	glairy	*ars, sil*
	of curdled milk	*nat m,* **sil**
	offensive smelling	arn, **ars,** bell, *bry, led,* merc, **nux v, sep**
	sour smelling	*ars, bell,* bry, *cimic,* gels, *hep,* ign, *merc, nat m,* nux v, **puls,** sep
	yellow	arn, *ars,* bry, *coloc,* merc
Sensation of a stone in the stomach		acon, arn, **ars, bry,** coloc, ign, *merc,* nat m, nux v, puls, *rhus t,* sep, sil
	after eating	*ars,* **bry,** nat m, **nux v,** *puls,* rhus t
Diarrhoea	after alcohol	ars, lach, **nux v**
	after anger	acon, ars, bry, **coloc,** *nux v*

	from bad news	*gels*
	during chill	ars, nux v, puls, rhus t
	after cold drinks	**ars,** bell, *bry, hep, puls, rhus t,* sep, *sil*
	during teething	*acon, ars, bell, coloc, gels, hep,* ign, *merc, sep,* **sil**
	> eating	*hep*
	with excitement	*gels*
	after fright	acon, **gels,** ign, *puls*
	after eating fruit	acon, **ars, bry, coloc,** lach, **puls**
	after eating sour fruit	lach
	in hot weather	*acon, ars, bell,* **bry**, lach, ,merc, *nat m*
	after ice cream	**ars,** bry, *puls*
	> lying on the abdomen	coloc, rhus t
	before menstruation	**lach,** *sil*
	during menstruation	ars, bry, nux v, *puls,* sil
	after milk	ars, bry, **sep,** *sil*
	< standing	ars, bry, ign
	excoriating	*arn,* coloc, hep, *ign,* lach, *merc, nat m,* nux v, *puls, sep*
	with tenesmus	**ars,** cimic, *coloc, merc*
	with pain after stool	ars, *bell, ign,* lach, **merc,** *nat m,* **puls,** *rhus t*
	with constant urging	arn, ars, bry, *ign,* **merc,** nat m, nux v, ruta
	with streaks of blood	arn, bry, *coloc,* led, **merc,** nux v, puls
	green stool	*acon, ars, bell,* bry, **coloc,** gels, *hep,* **merc, nat m,** *nux v,* **puls,** *rhus t, sep*
	lienteric stool	*arn,* **ars, bry,** *coloc,* hep, lach, *rhus t, sil*
	with mucus	acon, *arn, ars, bell, bry,* cimic, *coloc, hep,* ign, **merc, nux v, puls,** *rhus t, ruta,* sep, *sil*
Smell	cadaverous	**ars, lach**, *rhus t, sil*
	rotten eggs	*ars,* hep
	sour	*arn,* bell, *coloc,* **hep, merc,** sep, sil
	watery stool	arn, *ars,* bell, *coloc, hep, lach,* **merc, nat m, nux v, puls,** rhus t, sep, *sil*

Putting it all together

Here are some more little cases to have fun with. Once again you might like to cover up my comments until you have worked things out for yourself.

1. Unusually the patient had some beer with a celebratory meal. Now she feels nauseous and is salivating unnaturally. She is even developing a headache and simply could not face eating anything.

   Well, this is a simple acute with a clear exciting cause so you have three remedies to start with: *Bryonia*, *Lachesis* and *Nux vomica*. The salivation is very unusual so should stop and make you hesitate, then point to *Nux vomica*. The other three symptoms do not help you to discriminate unless there is a fuller symptom with Time, Location, Sensation and Modality. You might get these by asking more about the headache, but you are happy to give a *Nux vomica*. The 6th potency should be sufficient to help the liver cope with the beer!

2. During a headache, the patient suddenly develops a nausea whilst eating. This is much worse after forcing down some food.

   Again, not a very big case. You could get more symptoms from the headache but luckily you have a keynote of *Ruta* in nausea suddenly on eating, < after eating. Add to this that the nausea appears during a headache and you have a good case to give the remedy *Ruta* in a 6th potency. You would only go up to a 30th potency if the patient were low in vitality because of poor habits, and therefore slow to respond to the stimulation of a remedy. After the remedy, expect further developments as it is used to raise vitality by clearing out unwanted toxins.

3. After a heavy meal the patient developed a sensation of a weight in the stomach. Now, a few hours later this has led to diarrhoea of a watery nature with a horrible pong of rotten eggs. He has what is called a 'weak' digestion with a tendency to react to food. Does this explain why he is such a picky eater?

   The symptoms are very clear here. The weight in the stomach can be translated as a stone. After eating limits us to six remedies, whilst the watery diarrhoea further cuts down to five. When we add the rubric of the rotten egg smell we are left with only one remedy. However, since this last is a keynote we could have gone straight to that rubric where *Arsenicum* represents with a high value.

   The added information of the reactive digestion system and the patient's fastidiousness can only lead us to *Arsenicum*. Had we caught the case at the sensation level, we might only have needed a 6th potency but now it has advanced to the dysfunction level, even if eliminative, it may be better to give a single dose of the 30th potency. Remember, Homoeopathy always acts better in the single dose so it is better to give a potency appropriate to the amount of energy needed.

4. After eating fruit the patient has a bad case of diarrhoea that burns the anus on passing, leaving pain that continues on after the stool. On inspection, the food is discovered to be undigested (lienteric). Even though it was fruit that was eaten, the smell is of rotten flesh (cadaverous). The patient is very distressed.

   There are not many remedies with that distinct smell and even fewer of those are worse after eating fruit so we have only two remedies to choose from: *Arsenicum* and *Lachesis*. Both of these have burning pain which continues after the stool but in your repertory only *Lachesis* would describe this as excoriating. Since both remedies have lienteric stools, the differentiation is very subtle, especially as excoriating can be seen as rawness that burns. The way in which the patient is distressed might help confirm one or other remedy as *Arsenicum* will be so anxious they will think they are dying whilst might brood or become very nasty. Look for another symptom to clarify the case, or give a 6th potency of the faster acting *Arsenicum* then study its reaction. If the time taken to develop the symptom picture was longer, showing less vitality, I might reverse that and use the *Lachesis*. With a clearer symptom picture I would use the 30th potency in a single dose, *and take the case better next time*.

5. This lady always seem to have diarrhoea before menstruation. The stool is undigested but contains mucus too and may even smell sour on occasion. She is a thin, even emaciated, shy woman who is embarrassed to tell you her story.

   The Time is clear but it tells us that it is not a straightforward case but linked to the constitution so we may choose not to treat the diarrhoea as such, or it may indicate the constitutional remedy. The five remedies that appear under 'before menstruation' all have the possibility of mucus in the stool but only three have lienteric stools: *Arsenicum*, *Bryonia* and *Silicea*. Of these, only *Silicea* has the sour smell. Further *Silicea* is the shy one of the three. *Silicea* patients are often

described as emaciated and shy. For the acute episode, the 6th potency is probably sufficient especially as there is a weak slow response in the *Silicea* patient. On the constitutional level this might lead you to prescribe a 30th potency since the constitutional remedy is expected to work deeper and for longer. In an acute case, this may be too much activity, hence aggravation.

6. On holiday abroad, the woman has come down rapidly with something awful that started as yellow vomit but has continued with diarrhoea. There is much straining during the diarrhoea to produce a watery stool full of mucus and blood, and of course very smelly. She describes the smell eventually after much prodding as sour. She is very debilitated now so cannot answer much.

This is a common scene in many hotels overseas. It may be the heat or the unfamiliar food, or simply a 'bug'. We note she has started with yellow vomit that continues through the diarrhoea giving us two remedies: *Arsenicum* and *Mercurius*. The tenesmus (or straining) does not differentiate them and neither does the mucus in the stool. The blood in the stool points to *Mercurius*, as does the sour smell. These two remedies recur in holiday diarrhoea with little to distinguish them except something the chilliness of the *Arsenicum* with burning pains that need more heat. The *Mercurius* tends to sweat with the pain. The 6th potency might work in the case above, although it might need repeated on relapse of the symptoms. A single dose of the 30th potency might be a better choice since the coach will be waiting to move on next day.

I hope you have enjoyed these cases. If your watch out for Individuality, with clarity, precision and accuracy in your description of the symptoms, you should be able to get good results from using these little repertories.

READING

There are many books on the relationship with health, what we eat, and our environment. One of the earliest and still a significant read is *Silent Spring* by Rachel Carson.

THOUGHT TO PONDER

This individualising examination of a case of disease for which I shall only give in this space general directions, of which the practitioner will bear in mind only what is applicable for each individual case, demands of the physician nothing but freedom from prejudice and sound senses, attention in observing and fidelity in tracing the picture of disease.

Para 83, The Organon of the Rational Art of Healing
Samuel Hahnemann

LESSON 8   Menstrual Problems

Aims: To explore how dysfunction in the reproductive system manifests in acute ailments.
To explore the interaction of maintaining and exciting causes upon a susceptible constitution.
To show how remedies we have already studied may fit the symptom picture.
To study the remedies *Sepia, Cimicafuga*.

Keywords used:

congestion
Individuality
modality
Susceptibility
exciting cause

maintaining cause
affinity
concomitant
constitutional type

The Nature and Role of Menstruation

The female becomes capable of reproduction when she starts to ovulate in her teens. When the Pituitary Gland near the brain secretes a hormone (Follicle Stimulating Hormone, FSH) the egg in the ovary comes to fruition then is released into the Fallopian Tube where it passes along until it reaches the Uterus. If impregnated by a sperm, the egg will attempt to attach or embed itself in the lining of the Uterus, the Endometrium. If it succeeds it will grown into an embryo, the single cell dividing into many, becoming a foetus. The full gestation period is usually taken as nine calendar months – 39 weeks, or nine lunar cycles from conception.

More usually the egg is not fertilised so does not embed. The lining of the uterus which has grown soft and velvety in preparation to receive the egg is not needed now so it sloughs off leading to the 'period', or menstrual flow.

The whole process is carefully orchestrated by a series of hormones. The hormone that ripens the egg raises levels of oestrogen in preparation for pregnancy. It is the rising levels of progesterone that start the menstrual flow.

So what can go wrong?

CONGESTION

The cycle is interfered with in many ways. The most common today is congestion which can take two forms. The constitution may have a tendency to congest either because:

- it cannot handle fluid changes as the body prepares for pregnancy – the fullness of breasts increases, there is bloating in the abdomen and extremities, and dull bruised pain or cramps, or

- the liver is unable to remove excess oestrogen, now not needed, because it is already struggling with an overloaded system, often additional oestrogen from food. Liver congestion is usually indicated by constipation and/or congestive headaches before the period starts.

Either type of congestion is present in the constitutional symptom picture of many homoeopathic remedies. The first is usually indicative of a phlegmatic, or lymphatic, constitution whilst the second does arise in a more earthy constitution but can be seen to be a cumulative degeneration from a sluggish digestive system. Thus either type could have an exciting or maintaining cause; however, the clearest **individuality** in such a case is more usually the **modality**.

Congestion is further complicated because people today do not take nearly enough exercise. Exercise stimulates blood flow back to the abdominal organs (venous flow needs help from skeletal muscles contracting) and helps the reabsorption of fluid from intercellular spaces into veins and back to the kidneys. Lack of tone in the muscles means sluggish circulation so debris builds up, leading to poor skin tone and spots as well as further inhibiting the detoxification process of the liver, leading to more constipation. The constitutional weakness, the underlying fundamental cause, or miasm, thus is weakened further by lifestyle – the maintaining cause to the Homoeopath. So once again the initial interview with the Homoeopath involves checking diet and exercise habits to eliminate maintaining causes. Then constitutional homoeopathic treatment can strengthen predisposing weaknesses by removing **susceptibility** to exciting and maintaining causes. Constitutional treatment should give the Vital Force more energy to reverse the disease process bringing the expression of disturbance out from the *system* level.

EXERCISE AND THE MAINTAINING CAUSE

Lack of exercise and poor diet are maintaining causes that lower vitality allowing the constitutional weaknesses fuller expression. Attention here can remove much discomfort. I have come across a recent study that claims 1950s couples did the equivalent of 8 workouts each day. Yet some patients think a good programme is visiting the gym 2-3 times weekly. We live in a different world!

Alas, exercise is not just in the gym. How do we use our body hour by hour? Think of the continual movement of a shark or dolphin in the sea. Think of the chimpanzee's continual posture changes in the branches, not to mention the alertness to danger or food. Movement is a natural state of the body, our animal part. How do you use your body hour by hour?

Load bearing exercise throughout life leads to healthier bones and probably less osteoporosis. Many symptom pictures that occur at menopause point to poor calcium metabolism to the Homoeopath. It may be significant that the Tubercular [1] miasm throws out acutes most commonly at points of change in the calcium metabolism, such as teething (first and second), puberty (when there is a final spurt in growth of bones), pregnancy and menopause. Calcium balances iodine in the activity of the thyroid gland so where this metabolism is off balance we find the sluggish constitution and slow metabolism similar to that in the *Calcarea* patient. This is dysfunction rather than deficiency so today's remedy of calcium supplements is not only ineffective, it further disorders the metabolism. The Homoeopath is not impressed with the shopping basket analogy of health proposed when vitamins and minerals are added as compensations. Whilst this may be of use in extreme cases, ultimately the metabolism is not corrected in this way. Systems theory validates the gestalt model that the whole is greater than the sum of the parts.

Thus, movement internally and externally is fundamental to the totality or metabolism of the organism. At least 3-4 hours per day for ticking over, more for good health? Does this make you think of Qui Gong or Tai Chi?

DIET AND THE MAINTAINING CAUSE

Alas, diet often comprises of refined foods preserved with salt, sugar and fats with sugars and salt added to taste, along with other reconstituted tastes. Salt affects the natural fluid balance. Sugars affect the balance of blood sugar, plus fluid in some constitutions. Is it a wonder that diabetes is increasing at such a rate in our population? The swings of energy associated with the menses often lead to cravings before the period. Whilst the custom of eating no breakfast when blood sugar is low after fasting then eating much in the evening when the liver is starting to detoxify is extremely poor management that does not lead to efficiency or good health. To add to these problems, unnatural food also contains (as well as free radicals and non-antioxidants) xeno-oestrogens that give false hormonal signals **and** congest the liver, which controls levels of excretion of oestrogen. All of these are maintaining causes. Add coffee, which stimulates the liver, and releases more adrenaline which releases stored fat into the system, or tea, which paralyses smooth muscle causing lack of tone, and where are we? Did I mention alcohol and tobacco?

---

[1] The dominant miasm if we discount the cancer miasm.

Do not despair. To the Homoeopath each system is unique. We need to learn about our own system's weaknesses and strengths to achieve an optimum level of efficiency and health, i.e. each to their own poisons. No one diet or exercise plan will suit two people but attention to these two factors will improve most gynaecological problems of the nature discussed here.

> **EXERCISE**
>
> A little survey amongst your female friends and family members will show an amazing correlation between menstrual problems, amount of exercise and rich diet + overeating. Try to take a sample of 10 – 20. The table given below might be useful.
>
> What other questions might be useful?

Age	Problem	Amount exercise/day	Type of food eaten	Amount of food eaten

MENSTRUATION

The main problems here are pain, premenstrual syndrome and fluid retention. Irregularity and heavy flow should also be included as the one leads to problems with fertility and the last may lead to other problems such as anaemia. However, when we look at irregularity and heavy flow, we are not talking of an acute illness as in previous lessons. Put simply this is dysfunction in a *system* which has a rhythmic cycle. The menstrual period itself is not an illness, and if health is easy adaptation to change then there should be no discomfort and very little inconvenience – possibly just a bit more than having a bowel movement. It is important to put our expectations into proportion especially as this is a function that is grossly out of order in today's women. We might still be agreed that the cycle should last 28 days but how long should the bleeding take? My generation expect 4-5 days. Today it is common for young teenagers to experience 7 day periods. I would argue that this last is a sign of congestion and sluggish flow, just as obesity is now a common phenomenon of lack of exercise and poor diet.

Pain

As a teacher I found it really difficult that so many of my girl's class were absent with painful periods. As a Homoeopath, I am aghast that so many of these young women accepted 7 day periods, with pain and fluid retention, as *normal*.

There are two main types of dysmenorrhoea – spasmodic and congestive.

The **spasmodic** type is active and tense. There may be an emotional component as in *Ignatia* or *Lilium tigrinum* when the hormones are upset by *grief* or *disappointed love* (the unhappy end of a love affair) or in *Chamomilla* or *Staphisagria* when *anger* or *indignation* is the cause, **exciting cause**. The nature of the uterus is muscular going into spasm to deliver the child. It is sensitive to progesterone and postaglandins. An overbalance of progesterone causes excess spasm most commonly in the young girl so she has severe cramps on the first day of the period. *Nux vomica* and *Cimicafuga* can frequently be seen here as acute remedies of spasm. This type of dysmenorrhoea is expected to disappear in the mid 20s or with pregnancy as there is more oestrogen in the system. An exception may be when it accompanies membranous dysmenorrhoea, then the lining of the uterus comes off in such large and undissolved chunks which cannot be passed. The uterus goes into severe spasms notably before the flow starts – the flow being blocked. The remedy indicated may be *Lachesis* and it should come as no surprise that its keynote symptoms are also *bearing down pain, as if the contents of the abdomen would be expelled through the vagina.*[2]

We are talking of a pattern, not one incident but a recurrent trend. This shows it is not a simple acute as before. Indeed we will get nowhere treating such cases unless we treat the recurrent tendency that arises from constitutional weakness. To do this we must come to an understanding as to why the disease process manifests in the reproductive system. One answer is that it is complicated by the maintaining cause which interacts with the constitutional weakness, i.e. some constitutions are more prone to congesting factors because they already have a tendency to congest. In yet others the **affinity** is for the reproductive system so the exciting cause such as anger or disappointed love will upset the rhythm of the period – as in *Ignatia, Sepia, Lilium tigrinum, Natrum muriaticum, Pulsatilla, Chamomilla,* etc.

The **congestive** type is alas more common and represents the sluggish lymphatic flow mentioned above. It is greatly affected by poor fluid return or by liver congestion whether caused by maintaining cause or the constitution. See above. However yet another reason is a scrofulous constitution when it is an advanced manifestation of the tubercular miasm. Here the **affinity** is for the glands. The same girl will often have a history of colds and tonsillitis, glandular problems, even sinusitis where the inner tube becomes congested with mucus secretions. The ovum is slow to start its journey; the fallopian tubes may be congested. The pain is a dull ache before menstruation starts. The reproductive parts are more engorged than usual. This is accompanied in varying degrees by such symptoms of congestion as fluid retention and bloating, tender breasts, lethargy and constipation. It is expected to continue to menopause, getting worse with each successive pregnancy because of the link to a weakened calcium metabolism. Usually there is a strong reaction to contraceptive pills that further suppress the menstrual flow.

---

[2] This same remedy will be indicated later nearer menopause when the excessive contractions may be due to fibroids which is a structural change in a much further advanced disease process.

These are the types that would react strongly to contraceptive pills containing more or only oestrogen. The side effects of thrombosis and poor venous circulation in such constitutions would usually not be expected until much later in life, often in association with menopause.

Fluid Retention

As mentioned above, this is more common in the congestive type. The **time** and **location** when it occurs may indicate a characteristic or even **individualistic** pattern of a remedy. Remedies like *Sepia, Calcarea* and *Lycopodium* will bloat around the abdomen. In *Sepia* there is a tendency for the fluid to extend down the thighs. In *Calcarea, Bryonia, Pulsatilla* and *Silicea* the fluid retention is seen in tender breasts. In *Calcarea, Phosphorus* and *Sulphur* the hands and feet may be swollen and puffy. Headaches before the period in *Pulsatilla, Gelsemium* and *Natrum muriaticum* may be the result of fluid retention.

The table below puts much of the above theory into homoeopathic symptoms.

Type of Pain	Time	Location	Modality	Remedy
Aching		Lumbar Sacral		Gels Gels
Bearing down Burning				Lach, Sep Lach, Sep
Colicky		Abdomen		IGN, Mag p, Bry
Cramps		Abdomen Legs Uterine region	> bending double	Gels Gels Ign Coloc
Cutting		Through to loins		Hyos, Lach
Drawing		Forwards		Cham
Labour-like		Uterus and ovaries		Bell, Cham, Cimic, Mag p, Puls, Sep, Acon, Gels, Ign
Lacerating				Ign
Neuralgic		of distant parts		Cimic, Gels Gels
Pulsating				Cham
Shooting				Acon, Bell,
Stitching		To right of fundus uteri Naval -> uterus		Bry Acon Ipec
Tearing			Legs	Cham
Throbbing			Head	Lach

> **EXERCISE**
>
> There are a lot of gaps in the table. What can you fill in from your knowledge of the remedies so far?
>
> The following list of causation may help.

CAUSATION

This often contains both **Individuality** and **Susceptibility**.

Causation	
Anger	Bry, Cham, Coloc, Gels, Ipec, Lach, Nux v
Anxiety	Cimic, Ign
Alcohol	Bry. Calc, Gels, Led
Child-bearing	Cimic, Puls, Sep
Cutting Hair	Bell, Lach
Dentition	Cham
Disappointment	Gels
Disappointed Love	Cimic, Hyos, Ign, Lach
Discharges suppressed	Bry, Cham, Hyos, Led
Eating ices	Ars
Eating fruit	Ars
Eruptions suppressed	Bry, Calc, Ipec
Excitement	Calc, Cham. Phos
Exertion	Cimic, Rhus T
Fear	Acon, Phos
Fluids loss of	Calc, Chin
Fright	Acon, Ars, Bry, Calc, Cimic, Gels, Hyper, Ign, Lach
Grief	Ign, nat.
Heat	Acon, Gels
Jealousy	Hyos, Ign, Lach
Offence	Ign
Over-lifting	Calc, Rhus T
Use of Quinine	Ars, Ipec
Sweat suppressed	Calc
Tea	Cham
Tobacco	Ars, Ign

> **EXERCISE**
>
> If you have a copy of Kent's Repertory, it might be useful to colour the remedies above according to whether they aggravate **before, during** or **after the menses**.

CONCOMITANT SYMPTOMS

This is an interesting phenomenon that is invaluable to the Homoeopath. It is another kind of **individuality** that we see particularly in acutes that affects *systems*, but not exclusively. A concomitant symptom is one that accompanies another, unexpectedly and unrelated except in time. An example might be *painful urination with menses* as in *Cantharis*. There is no direct link and usually this would be treated as a different ailment with different medication by the Allopath. To the Homoeopath all is connected if only through the provings. In more physical ailments, there may be a common physiological cause. Then you must ask if these two always occur together with that cause. If the answer is no, and these two occur significantly in this patient, then you have something peculiar to that patient, a concomitant symptom.

Here are some examples:

Concomitant symptoms	
Anxiety with menstrual flow	Ign
Backache with menstrual flow	Sep
Conclusions with menstrual flow	Gels
Dropsy	Cham
Faintness with menstrual flow	Ign
Feels strange	Cimic
Headache	Bell, Cimic, Hyper, Ign
Haemorrhoids < menstrual flow	Lach
Heat in the head with menstrual flow	Ign
Nausea with menstrual flow	Hyper, Ipec
Photophobic	Ign
Temper < menstrual flow	Acon, Cham

PREMENSTRUAL TENSION

I have given a separate section to this as it takes many forms.

Congestion

The two types I have dealt with amply above. This is a build up of fluid and/or toxicity involving the efficiency of the liver as the detoxifying organ, heavily influenced by life style, interacting with the constitutional type.

Headaches

These are of two main types: the congestive **bilious** headache is related to congestion; the **migraine** brings in a nervous theme not necessarily separate from fluid retention in remedies like *Natrum muriaticum, Apis* and *Gelsemium*.

In the first type, bilious, we might consider remedies such as *Bryonia, Nux vomica*, even *Sepia* and *Pulsatilla* which both have portal vein stasis. All of these remedies have accompanying nausea and aggravation from heat. They have different degrees of reaction to motion. Although ultimately better for flow, *Bryonia* likes to be still and is severely aggravated by motion. *Nux vomica* and *Sepia* may aggravate from initial movement but are ultimately better on the go. Indeed *Sepia* is better for violent exertion at one stage – before it goes into abdominal sag. *Pulsatilla* is better for continued gentle motion, as long as it is not overheated.

The term 'migraine' is much bandied about. Truly it involves the nervous system but the nature of the head structure is such that some congestion, especially fluid but also toxic, strongly affects sensitive nerve tissue. *Apis* and *Gelsemium* are remedies where fluid congestion before the period can lead to severe migraine headaches, clumsy movements and loss of co-ordination of limbs and speech. In *Apis* the memory for words may be affected, even the behaviour.

Mood Swings and Behavioural Disturbance

This can be a frightening change of personality for the woman and her family. Congestive types such as *Pulsatilla* and *Sepia* may weep before the period for no reason. Sulkiness is found in other glandular types such as *Antimonium crudem, Baryta carbonicum, Silicea* as well as *Pulsatilla*. Remedies such as *Nux vomica, Lycopodium* and *Sepia* will get very angry before the period whilst others such as *Lachesis, Hyoscyamus and Pulsatilla* will get very jealous and spiteful if *Apis* is needed.

Amenorrhoea – no menstrual period

Usually the menstrual period starts about 11, 12, 13 years. In some constitutions (*Pulsatilla, Calcarea, Silicea*) the girl's body matures more slowly so it may be 15, 16 or even 17 years before the period starts. Constitutional treatment may speed up maturation but there is a bit more to it than having periods.

Puberty is an important growth point, which involves a shift in the Calcium metabolism as the body spurts to its adult height. If bone growth is too quick and spindly (think of seedlings), as in some *Phosphorus* patients, vitality is affected leaving the patient open to respiratory infections – pneumonia is common in the *Phosphorus* patient at this time if growth is too fast. Weight-bearing exercise is so important at this time to encourage healthy bone. Walk or run 2-3 hours/day at least. (All those 15 minutes add up.)

At puberty the young girl takes on the shape of a woman. Fat distribution changes, breasts develop. Marilyn Monroe was size 16 and weighed 11 stone, I am informed! The fat stores must reach a specific proportion before menstruation starts. If it falls below this level menstruation will stop – the gymnast and the ballet dancer are examples of super-fit girls who may not menstruate because there is not enough fat. In this day the anorexic or bulimic girl's fat levels may drop too low to menstruate. The fat and calcium metabolism meet in the thyroid function, which regulates metabolic rate, so lack of energy may be a general symptom of imbalance or the wrong balance. Constitutional remedies with an emotional content that might lead to emaciation or eating disorder are *Natrum muriaticum, Pulsatilla* and *Ignatia*.

In terms of diet, Vitamin E and the Essential Fatty Acids are essential to the formation of many hormones. These are found in seeds, wheatgerm, soybean oil, corn oil and safflower oil. Add a spoonful of mixed seeds and wheatgerm to breakfast muesli or lunchtime salads. Long term lack of protein causes inability to reabsorb fluid in the extremities.

Heavy Flow

The flow frequently gets heavier as the woman gets older, although this need not be the case. It is common in the lymphatic type of constitution that becomes congested – there is that word again. Usually the early periods are lighter often because no egg is released by the ovary at first so there is less oestrogen. This is less true of today's young women with their 7 day heavy periods, I suspect because of oestrogen in food. But, what is heavy? How long should a period last? Constitutions differ. In patients after treatment I aim for 4-5 days and do not expect heavy flooding or change of protection more than 6 hours. That must be only a guideline. Each generation seems longer and heavier. Why? Why don't they do medical research on this type of thing?

There are constitutional reasons but once again I put it down to too rich food, poor exercise, and sedentary occupation, all leading to congestion. There is much we can do to help ourselves.

Acne

I have put this teenager's nightmare in here because it usually starts with the flow of hormones. It arises in certain constitutional types the Homoeopath would call *Tuberculoid*. Basically the lymphatic system is congested as fat metabolism is compromised. The answer is therefore threefold:

- correct the hormone imbalance constitutionally
- cut the excessive intake of poly-saturated fats and/or balance the diet with poly-unsaturated fats
- stimulate the skin.

Correcting the hormonal balance is constitutional work to create a better health balance. Maintaining causes can be removed by increased flow lymphatically – exercise again.

Work on diet may be simple. Modern packaged food is full of salt, fats and sugar – eliminate it. Staple foods such as oats, wheat (bread), potatoes and rice contain slow release carbohydrates that nurture us throughout the day hence the old adage *breakfast like a king, lunch like a prince and dine like a pauper*. It is breakfast that gets us through the day. Overnight the liver detoxifies if it does not have a lot of food to digest. Sumo wrestlers eat in the evening to put on weight, I'm told!

So ... add fruit and vegetables to basic foods

do not eat after 6.00pm

if thirsty, when thirsty, drink water, not sugar

acknowledge stimulants as luxuries the body may not be able to afford so use accordingly and sparsely

cut down on all added sugar, salt and fats and dairy produce.

Dairy produce comes from specialised lymph glands called breasts that produce a specialised form of lymph, milk, which increases lymphatic congestion by its very nature. Besides cows have four stomachs so calves have different enzymes to humans to enable them to digest cow's milk.

To stimulate the skin, plenty of bracing fresh air whilst you are walking to work or school is by far the cheapest way with the benefit of being weight-bearing exercise. Of course, before you leave, you will have had a shower finished with a quick rinse of cold water to zap the skin.

And if you have forgiven me for all that, we will move on.

USEFUL REMEDIES

Belladonna	Violent spasms. Rush of blood to the head with throbbing headache. The abdomen is hot, distended and tender to touch. There is restlessness with an over-sensitivity of all the senses. The pulse is full and hard.
Bryonia	Distension of the abdomen and colic. They may describe a heavy feeling like a stone in the abdomen. Usually there is constipation before the period. Touchy and irritable. They want to be left alone and to lie still. Often with a congestive headache beforehand and swelling that extends to the extremities especially in rheumatic types. The pulse is hard and hurried. There may be nosebleeds at the time of menstruation, even instead of menstruation.
Cantharis	This is another remedy of membranous dysmenorrhoea but is very different from *Lachesis* in that there is burning pain in the vulva and ovary, an itchy vagina and painful urination.

Chamomilla   There is such a sensitivity to pain that it is unbearable and drives them to despair. The spasms can be identified by the numbness that accompanies them. The discharge smells foetid. They are spiteful, peevish and restless. They will hate to be looked at. There may be heavy night sweats, wind and indigestion.

Lachesis   When not membranous, this type is congestive with a build-up of fluid giving a sensitive and distended abdomen. They do not want any clothes around the abdomen. They are sluggish but not relieved by resting. Indeed they are much worse in the morning after sleep. They are also sensitive to heat and are worse after eating. The extremities are often blue and cold. The head may be hot with congestive dull aching pains. The menstrual pains are bearing down – the more congested, the more severe until they will describe it as if the contents of the abdomen were being expelled. It is a remedy of prolapse.

Magnesium Phosphoricum   This is a useful remedy of spasm. The pains are described as colicky. There may be heat in the abdomen and wind. They are better for heat and bending double which distinguishes it from *Nux vomica*.

Nux vomica   This is another remedy of spasm but also represents the congestive liver type so constipation is usually a feature before the period but not accompanied by fluid retention. The abdomen may be distended but if so it will be wind. The pains are colicky. There will be sensitivity to food and heat so they will not eat. This type improves with exercise and fasting beforehand to lower the congestion. They are extremely irritable, especially sensitive to noise and can be violent but are more likely to curse and swear.

Pulsatilla   The presentation here varies with age as congestion increases. In the young girl the period is easily offset by getting the feet wet. It is often late or irregular and tends to flow more in the day when they are active. The pain may be intense when they are younger. Later the build-up will be more prominent with fluid retention and painful breasts especially on the right side, and cold extremities. They are often chilly. The pain may be better with a hot water bottle. This type tend to comfort eat sweets.

Remedies

Sepia

This is called the Washerwoman remedy after one of Hahnemann's patients. She came to him all worn out with the effort of earning a living and keeping her family going. She did not come back because she was too busy and Hahnemann found her at the ford doing her washing having got enough sustenance from the remedy to get on with her life.

Sepia is a busy-bee, > occupied. Picture this woman! You are bound to know one at least. Why is she always on the go? She is *dutiful* and has an ideal to which she works. This makes her *fastidious* and fussy, hard working, but she is the type who will see her surroundings (or her job in modern women who also work outside the home) as an extension of herself and therefore take any intrusion personally as an attempt to spoil her, an attack on her very existence. She can easily be mistaken for an *Arsenicum* patient at this point. She will continually attempt to 'correct' her space, injecting herself more and more into it, controlling it by telling others it is her person they are tampering with. In this she is like *Natrum muriaticum* – both have an enormous area of personal space around them.

Sepia defends her space actively by *nagging* or by intense *irritability*. She stretches herself so much in her efforts that health is affected as she does not have enough energy to go around. Her changed behaviour will show this first then her body will show the typical *sag* which is usually taken as the essence of *Sepia*. At first, she does not last through the afternoon then she becomes increasingly exhausted then indifferent.

The remedy is taken from the special sac in the cuttlefish where it is stored. The animal uses this 'ink' to squirt a dark cloud into the sea around it. From this cloud it is invisible to friend or foe, to its predators and its prey, and so the *Sepia* patient uses its space to create a facade to hide the real person. When she is worn down and exhausted she retreats into a cloud. First there may be aimless aggression, prickliness, (*how many husbands know it is that time of the month?*) then she withdraws and isolates herself. In this sullen depression she is beyond the reach of others, *indifferent to loved ones*. If the withdrawal is very serious she will hide, refusing to open the door or will go to the other side of the street to avoid those she knows. She does not want them to see her because she is not herself.

Sepia has a close affinity to the condition of the congested liver that cannot deal with oestrogen excretion. Thus, its most common modalities are < *menses,* < *pregnancy,* < *menopause*. Her metabolism is sluggish, increased by portal vein stasis. Her abdomen is swollen and pendulous pulling her spine out of alignment so backache is a common feature especially before the menses and during pregnancy. In the worst cases there are piles and varicose veins worse on the *left side* as *Sepia* symptoms go *from left to right*, as in its acute remedy *Lachesis*. Her headaches are of the congestive type, a dull pain *over the left eye* worse in the morning and better as the day goes on, but worse when the menstrual flow is scanty.

The congested *Sepia* is > *violent exertion,* even the headache is better exertion. She is known to enjoy dancing – you might see this as jogging or the gym in today's executive. The congestion of the period is seen also when it is prolonged and clotted, and tails off in a *brown discharge*. She may be prone to get severe migraines on the left side with *zig zag vision. Natrum muriaticum* is the only other remedy with this last symptom. Like *Natrum muriaticum,* this remedy is averse to sexual intercourse. Whilst *Natrum muriaticum* is often described as frigid, *Sepia* will have low sex drive; she *cannot be bothered* or is even < *after coition* and she can have a headache! There may be little time in her busy schedule for intimacy. At her worse, she is even averse or *indifferent to her children*.

The sag in the abdomen tends to diverticular disease, more commonly diagnosed as Irritable Bowel Syndrome today. Then the swelling and congestion in the abdomen leads to a keynote symptom, *as if the contents of the abdomen would be expelled through the vagina*. This is the *Sepia* that *desires acid foods*, particularly vinegar, to give tone to the digestive system. The same *Sepia* is *worse for beer*. In her weak state, she tends to faint. She has *nausea at the sight and smell of food,* like *Arsenicum*. This is most evident in pregnancy so it comes as no surprise that this remedy is frequently used in pregnancy.

It is also used for a tendency to miscarry in the fifth month, or the seventh month, as the uterus is too weak to carry the child. In the pregnancy we will find backache, varicose veins and piles and later, if the hormones are slow to regain balance, there may be Post Natal Depression when she is indifferent to her child and just cannot be bothered. Her partner may be patient but she does not regain her sex drive.

The sensation of *Sepia* is *hollowness* or *of a ball*. In the nausea, there is a sensation of a ball in the stomach or of a ball rising up the oesophagus. Remember the sac or bladder that contained the ink in the cuttle fish? *Sepia* is a remedy of hollow organs, viz. stomach, uterus, prostate bladder and gall bladder. It is remedy of cystitis that has *burning pains that shoot up,* as the pain of the piles burns and shoots up.

The stomach has the sensation of emptiness or a lump and frequently there is a hiatus hernia – a common symptom at menopause especially with gall stones in the gall bladder, i.e. little round balls. The stool is knotty with the sensation of a lump in the anus that does not go away after going to the toilet. It is a remedy of the prostate when enlarged. The uterus is prone to fibroids.

Sepia is a very common remedy at time of menopause especially when metabolism slows down. There may be under-active thyroid. Flushes of heat upwards and even palpitations with heat or the slightest exertion is a common symptom when there is congestion. Backache, migraines on the left side, hiatus hernia, nausea, indifference, heavy prolonged bleedings and fibroids may complete the picture. The individuality is the heat moving upwards, the burning pains moving upwards, sensations of lumps or emptiness, left sidedness. Another symptom of the mature woman that relates back to the cuttle fish is the pigmentation often called liver spots that appear in later life. *Sepia* is a sycotic remedy that grows things like warts and moles, also made up of the pigment melanin.

Cimicifuga

Also called *Actaea Racemosa*, it is a remedy of spasm very similar to *Nux vomica* so it is important to differentiate it. Another name, Squaw Root, shows it came to us from the American Indians who knew its use for female problems.

Its **affinity** is for muscles so if we say it is also used as a remedy of rheumatism you will begin to see the type of constitution we are working with when we use this remedy. There is a lack of flow in muscular tissue so lactic acid builds up after excessive exercise giving rise to soreness and stiffness. As in *Ruta*, the eyeballs can be affected so they ache after the dancing, especially if this social occasion involves much alcohol – the symptom picture is now also similar *Ledum*. The **modalities** are those of the rheumatic: > warmth that improves movement, > continued movement, > open air; the rheumatic pains are particularly < damp and < at night. The muscular aches cause the patient to toss and turn in bed at night so sleep is not refreshing. This further stresses bringing on depression with weepiness – *a sensation as if a heavy, black cloud had settled all over her and enveloped her head, so that all is darkness and confusion.* Is it any wonder she thinks she will go insane?

Cimicifuga is one of a group of remedies where the affect on muscle includes heart and uterus, in acupuncture the extra-ordinary vessel, the solid organ (heart) and its hollow counterpart (uterus). Thus, we must look to see where the Vital Force compensates or holds the disturbance away from these vital organs. Rheumatism is usually a defence of the heart as we will see in the next lesson. The depressive rheumatics are particularly 'heart' types in so far as there is a loss of spontaneity and the joy of life; they become disconnected from others. Lippe quotes that 'in all her mental symptoms there is a lack of coherence'. This is a bit further than the indifference of *Sepia* and more like the nervous disorganisation of *Natrum muriaticum* and *Apis*. Indeed we are told that *Cimicifuga* also acts through the nerves. There are nervous twitches, spasms and convulsions *< menstruation.* One of the signs of nervous involvement is the presence of many sensations, so there is no simple headache for her – it has the **sensation** *as if the top would fly off* which also contains the **Essence** of lack of coherence. If you think of what we mean by a nervous type, they think the world is out to get them, they are jumpy, they are sensitive and hyperactive – the word 'hysterical' is often used here. And, just as 'hysteria' comes originally from the Greek for womb, activity of the uterus, such as menstruation, is the weak point or **Susceptibility** of this remedy, hence why it is seen so commonly as a woman's remedy. Turned inward it becomes melancholia or depression even Post Natal Depression when the uterus is the muscle disordered.

On the sensation level there is pain beneath the left breast – *which is to the uterus what pain in the shoulder is to the liver,* i.e. referred pain. There is much uterine pathology including prolapse *during menstruation,* bleeding between periods with pains running down from the hips into the thighs, false labour pains and even miscarriage in the third month. It is a remedy of over-excitability during labour with severe spasmodic pains, *aggravated by noise* and characterised by *shivers in the first stage of labour.*

The spasmodic nature is found not only in muscular action but also in the suddenness of onset of symptoms – sudden sinking in the pit of the stomach, the heart suddenly ceases during uterine problems, colicky pains that bend them double after passing a stool, convulsions *with menstruation*, chorea-type movements with rheumatism, and of course cough. As in many rheumatic remedies, there is a cough on the first level of acute. This is a dry short cough that starts as a tickle and is worse speaking or trying to speak – very similar to *Phosphorus*.

In speaking of this remedy, I have mentioned many other remedies. I have not done this before to keep it simple but there are over 2000 homoeopathic remedies with much similarity and overlap and yet, to get best results, we have to prescribe accurately. The Homoeopath matches the symptom picture of the patient accurately to that of the remedy using especially **Individuality** and **Susceptibility,** those two magic words without which a homoeopathic prescription would not be very useful. In bringing in the other remedies here, you can see just how accurate the Homoeopath can be, or has to be! It is < *menstruation* or menstruation as an **exciting cause** that has caused me to add this remedy to this section.

LET US LOOK AT A FEW CASES

Case A

This patient has a history of grief (**Exciting cause**) with several miscarriages over a period of 10 years. She has a tendency to fluid imbalance giving rise to migraines with zig zag vision and rheumatism with swollen left knee and hip. After each miscarriage she has increasing fluid imbalance, first headache before menses now rheumatism too.

The constitutional remedy is *Natrum muriaticum* and this will access the exciting cause and has **affinity** for fluid imbalance.

The acute remedy *Sepia* is used for fluid build-up before the period leading to left sided migraine with zig zag vision, swollen breasts and abdomen – as if the contents would fall out through the vagina, indifference to children and irritability with partner before period. Confirming the acute remedy is nausea with headache < at the sight of food.

So how do we use the *Sepia*? When indicated is too late. We need to catch it at the start of the build-up and we need to affect the dysfunction level so the 30^h potency is given at ovulation each cycle until relief sets in. The constitutional remedy is given once only in high potency during the amelioration phase after the period, and then overall progress is carefully assessed.

Case B

The patient is a young girl leading a sedentary life whilst studying for exams. Her confidence is poor and she comfort eats to cope. There is lymphatic congestion of breasts before the menstrual period plus distended abdomen with constipation and nausea relieved by a hot water bottle. Note, that you see here the **general modality** of < before menses and the **particular modality** of abdomen dysfunction > heat.

This is an acute condition of a constitutional remedy. Here we have its **predisposition** lack of confidence; and her adaptation pattern, comfort eating. The **affinity** of the remedy is for the glands and lymphatic system including breasts and ovaries. The remedy also affects visceral muscle which swells causing constipation (and sometimes diarrhoea). The same remedy is sensitive to hormonal change (**general modality**) which tends to congest and slow down fluid exchange.

So the remedy *Pulsatilla* covers the **predispositions** and the acute situation of **affinity** and **modality**. There is further the **Individuality** of comfort eating. We can use *Pulsatilla 30* to relieve the fluid congestion symptoms and act constitutionally on the cause to help her cope better. Whilst we might give one dose during this current period, we will try to give a higher more constitutional dose before the next period.

Case C

This patient smokes and drinks heavily (**maintaining cause**). Her skin has the earthy hue of someone whose liver is compromised and she suffers from constipation if she does not have bran flakes each morning.

Before the menstrual period starts, for 1-2 days, she has violent abdominal cramps that are immediately increased with a hot water bottle (**modality**) but it brings on the flow and helps in the longer term. She is also better when she exercising more in the week before the period. If allowed to build up she has bilious headaches and nausea (**concomitant symptom**). The pain is on the top of her head as if there was a brick weighing her head down (**Individuality**). It is worse lying down and any sensory input especially noise (**Individuality** and **modality**). Noise turns her irritability into rage when she curses and feels generally murderous (**Individuality**)!

This is a more acute case of spasmodic dysmenorrhoea created by a maintaining cause of alcohol and tobacco. Thus, while we might choose to use a 6th potency of *Nux vomica* repeated every half hour until relief sets in, we would advise on change of diet and habit. We choose the repeat dose to relieve slowly the congested liver. A higher potency would aggravate severely.

EXERCISE

Can you identify the prescribing symptoms in the above cases?

I have made it quite a bit easier by telling you the remedies!

READING

There are many good books out of late with a more natural approach to women's ailments. Miranda Castro's book *Mother and Baby* will give you more conditions and more homoeopathic remedies.

THOUGHT TO PONDER

In accordance with this fact it is undeniably shown by all experience that the living human organism is much more disposed and has a greater liability to be acted on and to have its health deranged by medicinal powers, than by morbific noxious agents and infectious miasms; or in other words, that the morbific noxious agents possess a power of morbidity deranging man's health that is subordinate and conditional, often very conditional; while medicinal agents have an absolute unconditional power, greatly superior to the former.

Para 33, The Organon of the Rational Art of Healing
Samuel Hahnemann

LESSON 9   Rheumatism and Arthritis

Aims: To demonstrate acute treatment in a degenerative disease.
To define what is meant by these disease labels.
To understand the nature of Rheumatism as a disease of circulation, of congestion and over-acidity.
To study the exciting cause as a stress (or modality) on the constitution.
To explore how lifestyle accelerates degenerative disease, or can help you get the best out of your constitution.

Keywords:
degenerative disease
particular symptoms
indicating symptoms
direction of cure
palliation

A Disease of Old Age?

These are two diseases that are expected in old age. When we define old age, or if you have an image of an old person, it usually involves the bent wasted frame with pain and discomfort that we call arthritic. Are you looking forward to the time when you will be bent and in pain? Can you picture yourself old? They used to say that if gynaecologists were women many common female ailments would have solutions by now! Here is an interesting situation of the inevitable that happens to a powerless group with a small voice. Do we have to look forward to rheumatism and arthritis?

Previously it was seen as a degenerative disease, wear and tear or worn out tissue so the only treatment is generally pain relief or anti-inflammatory drugs. *(Note the change to the present tense, i.e. nothing has changed in practice.)* The only advance in arthritis appears to be in replacing joints artificially. In rheumatism there is another understanding of the body's role in inflammation – see below. Only the Naturopaths saw that these two could be abolished, and that through nutrition. The fact that such illnesses are now recognised and accepted in younger and younger people must raise questions.

What is Rheumatism and Arthritis?

These two are banded together but what is the difference? Rheumatism is often seen to progress into Arthritis. Arthritis when it occurs in younger people is often seen as a drug side-effect, e.g. from the use of steroids.

Usually when we talk of Arthritis we mean Osteo-arthritis, a degenerative disease where the cartilage at the end of bones is worn so becomes rough especially with repeated use. Movement is affected, becoming difficult and painful. There may be calcium deposits irritating the surrounding tissue when the joint is moved so giving rise to swelling and pain. Eventually the joint becomes less flexible, hard and knotty and movement is painful. Also, where the tendons contract the joint may be distorted. Some joints are more susceptible than others, so knees and hips are common sites because they carry the weight of the whole body; the shoulders may be a common site in the sedentary scriber who sits hunched over a desk; the fingers are common in the pianist, the feet in the ballet dancer. Note that the Naturopath would ask why the body is not healing.

Osteoporosis is different from arthritis and not necessarily related. This disease affects the formation of healthy bone so in the afflicted person the bones are thinner and more brittle. Thus they may break more easily or simply fail to support the skeleton. It is commonly associated with hormonal changes – these days menopause – and with the prolonged use of glucocorticoids such as prednisone. Any factors that affect the metabolism of calcium, Vitamin D and protein may contribute. And the Naturopath? She might ask how the bones were being used and attempt in the early stages to question lifestyle. For example, is there a link between our increasingly sedentary lifestyle and therefore little use of weight-bearing bones?

Rheumatoid Arthritis is different again. It is an auto-immune disease creating inflammation in joints, especially small joints such as the fingers and toes, but also the spine in some. It progresses to other joints of course. The mechanism is more destructive. Cartilage is eroded by enzymes then as fibrosis sets in, the joints becomes fixed, or ankylosed. As the muscles atrophy, the tendons are stretched and the unstable joint is pulled out of shape. As a systemic disease there are further symptoms that cause fatigue, low grade fever and anaemia.

Gout manifests as hard swollen joints when uric acid crystals are deposited, usually due in acute situations such as dietary indiscretions in individuals with impaired kidney excretion. There may be many causes of the latter including kidney disease.

So, what happened to rheumatism? Like fibrositis, it is no longer a legitimate diagnosis. It has become a factor, rheumatoid factor (RF), an antibody, causing swelling and stiffness in joints. In large joints it is called synovitis and is seen as an early form of arthritis. The terms 'acute rheumatism' or 'rheumatic fever' are retained to explain sudden swelling resulting after injury in particular but also after infection, or drug reaction. Thus, we can say Rheumatism is associated with inflammation and circulatory disturbances. Gran would recognise this and it is this that is spoken of in old homoeopathic books.

We commonly speak of a symptom picture, or even a diathesis, that involves muscular stiffness, especially the morning after excessive exercise or a soaking. The Homoeopath would call this a rheumatic constitution. Those sensitive to such changes will talk of getting chilled after sweating (**exciting cause**), leading to fever and muscular stiffness.

The athlete will take care not to catch a chill after exertion, even the racehorse is walked until it cools down after the race. Those of you into aerobic exercise will know to warm up first to stop muscles going into spasm, or cramps – the swimmer is advised not to swim after a meal as they might then be more liable to cramp especially if the water is cold – and then after exercise, you need to move the muscles slowly so they do not cool down too quickly.

We are talking about **circulation** and redistribution of heat and the effect of sudden chilling on muscles. Rheumatism is about muscles, rather than bones – **affinity**. The Naturopath might speak of congestion in this regard. In the acute situation there is a lack of flow so lactic acid is built up as a product of metabolism – this is why rheumatism is seen as a disease of 'overacidity' by the Naturopath. As in gout, acute bouts may arise after over acid food, or anger! It is because of the acid congestion that there is stiffness on first movement, stiffness first thing in the morning > as the day goes on.

Later in life, the muscles become weakened and may 'give way'. Technically, we are speaking here of a modality that overloads, or pushes the constitution further, and it may be so in very debilitated types who are already showing their symptoms and are then aggravated by the modality.

In other types, when the symptoms are not apparent, the exciting cause seems to bring out the symptom picture, or an acute bout of illness. It is not necessary to split hairs here. The information is useful in choosing a potency. The case with the modality may need a smaller potency, perhaps repeated, whilst the case with the exciting cause may need a single dose of a higher potency such as the 30th. In allopathic terms the first case is more chronic; in homoeopathic terms the disease process is further advanced in the case with the modality so we need to go slower to match the lesser energy.

Rheumatic fever is an acute illness that causes inflammation in muscles due to Streptococcal infection. In more serious cases it affects heart muscle and may be identified many years later by its effect on heart valves causing heart murmurs as it shortens the tendons opening the mitral valve in particular.

A HOMOEOPATHIC INTERPRETATION

In Homoeopathy, we take into consideration the symptom pattern rather than the disease, since we recognise only one disease, the disturbance of the Vital Force's ability to maintain harmony. The symptoms tell us how deeply the disturbance has penetrated the Vital Force's activity and this in turn determines the potency used and case management. To find the indicated remedy that will restore the Vital Force to health, we need to identify what is individual in the symptom picture to match closely the Similimum. There are no routine prescriptions in Homoeopathy. Always we treat the individual.

In Rheumatism and Arthritis, we are looking at the manifestation of deep disturbance that has occurred over a period of many years. What is now visible as symptoms is not just the attempt of the Vital Force to cure; at this stage in the disease process the symptoms also represent the products of the pathological process and a point of balance or containment of a degenerative disease that will end in death if nothing else intervenes. Therefore, cure is a long term proposition that will go through as many stages as it took the disease to get to this point. In persuading the organism to heal, we need to create more energy and increase vitality by lowering the toxic levels. Like the Naturopath, we can attend to the maintaining causes of diet and exercise but, as Homoeopaths, we can be more proactive with our remedies.

I will not deal here with Rheumatic Fever that needs skilled prescription of acute remedies.

Osteo-arthritis, for the time being, I will see as a progression of Rheumatism, as it was once seen. It also will benefit from attention to the maintaining cause.

THE ACUTE SYMPTOM PICTURE

Muscles may be stiff and sore form unaccustomed use. This will come under the heading of *Sprains and Strains* requiring remedies such as *Arnica* and *Rhus toxicodendron* as already mentioned in Lesson 2. In this Lesson, I want to go deeper into a certain constitutional type who is prone to muscular aches on exposure. The main **exciting causes** of the rheumatic type are *getting soaked* or *becoming chilled especially after overheating* or simply *over-exposure to cold*. Getting soaked reminds us also that the rheumatic type can tell that the weather is about to change. They are sensitive to the increasing humidity in the air or to the lowered atmospheric pressure before a storm. Thus, the exciting cause may be an **Individuality** that helps us to identify the remedy.

Because the stiffness is caused by slow drainage of lactic acid from the tissues, the most common **modality** is *worse first movement and better continued movement*. This symptom is present in many acute rheumatic remedies. Other modalities may thus point to **Individuality.** Note that **Susceptibility** here is the underlying constitutional type that has reached a particular stage in the disease process. The word *particular* is here significant as indeed this symptom picture is of particulars in the sense that this is the level of adaptation of the Vital Force. The patient will come to us with disturbance visible as **particular** symptoms. This is the level at which the disturbance of the Vital Force is contained. The processes are physiological and may produce **General** symptoms when they affect the sweating patterns, for example.

In treating sudden onset of symptoms after exposure to the exciting cause, it may be prudent to use one only dose of the 30th potency recognising the assault on the Vital Force and returning the adaptation to the previous level. There may be expected a short aggravation and quick resolution of the flare-up overnight.

MANAGING THE CHRONIC CASE

This is an important subject since in these cases the stage of degeneration is often well-developed, thus involving pain and immobility. There are three stages of disease to the Homoeopath: sensation, dysfunction and structural change. In advanced stages of this illness, there is structural change which needs a great deal of energy to reverse. Since a sudden blast will destroy the integrity of the patient and anyway the disease has progressed insidiously, cure will take much time. This is an example of the type of illness where the Homoeopath will not use high potencies but low potencies even in repeat doses. There are ways of managing the treatment. It may be best to use plussed remedies or even LM potencies as there is a limited return repeating the dose – it is even possible to enter the second phase of the remedy's action with much repetition.

Whichever method is chosen I strongly advise that you select **indicating symptoms** and watch these carefully for **direction of cure**. Whilst it might be relevant to palliate such a case, especially in the very elderly, the Homoeopath will still watch the action of the remedy carefully because **palliation** is a balance between the acute and chronic expression of the symptoms and not cure.

Managing the chronic case must involve attention to the maintaining causes to lower the toxic load, whatever aggravates the condition. There are excellent diets for arthritis that involve removal of acid-creating foods and increase in the body's alkalinity. It is interesting that Nature provides so we find that such foods grow naturally in wet climates that are more liable to create such conditions, e.g. oats, temperate fruits such as apples.

One group of foods universally 'bad' for arthritis and rheumatism is the *Solanacaea* that create heat of the irritable kind and are often remedies of rashes, urticarea and allergic response – tomatoes, aubergines, courgettes, potatoes, peppers of all kinds. One exception to this is the remedy *Dulcamara* that demonstrates the homoeopathic Law of Similars – see below. One of the more acute remedies of the group *Belladonna* might be a remedy of Rheumatic Fever. See the diet following.

Exercise that involves movement is very useful to encourage flow and drainage, thus relieving congestion. Massage may be invaluable in certain cases to stimulate blood circulation to affected parts, the *particulars*, and as lymphatic drainage may do much to improve the later oedemas of rheumatism or the predisposing conditions, i.e. the stiffness has less chance to develop if fluid exchange is up to scratch. However, the best massage is internal and I encourage such types to take up Tai Chi and Qi Gong. The slow flowing movement in these two practices are ideal for rheumatic types in promoting flow of body fluid whilst Hatha Yoga is unsurpassed for keeping joints flexible and avoiding the contraction of arthritis.

However, both these ailments demonstrate the truth of how we use and look after the body. Muscles and skeletal bones were make for a purpose and are healthiest whilst fulfilling that purpose. I encourage patients not to overdo things but to develop a lifestyle in which they have a happy relationship with their body.

How do they use their body from hour to hour through the day? What does it enable them to do? How do they need it to perform? How do they enjoy it? An hourly, daily relationship is infinitely better than a workout at the gym three times a week! The very best exercise is probably regular walking.

By studying the patient's miasm, the Homoeopath can predict the pattern of disease likely long before it is manifest. There are some exercises following.

Lesson 9

SOME REMEDIES FOR SHORT TERM MANAGEMENT

Whilst these remedies are most useful in managing the discomfort of Rheumatism or Arthritis, first ask what you hope to achieve by using them. Set clear goals and choose indicating symptoms that will help you monitor progress.

Rhus toxicodendron   This remedy is specific to ligaments, tendons and muscles and has the common modalities *< first movement better continued movement, > heat, > massage, < cold, wet conditions, < before a storm.* The importance of movement comes out in their restlessness, they have to keep moving. They cannot sleep because they have to keep moving, or they *dream of exertion* and wake exhausted. *Rhus toxicodendron* has an affinity for the histamine reaction of mast cells so its keynotes are *itch* and *oedema*. The itch is mainly in the early stages where skin problems are associated but in later stages it will produce numbness and prickling, *as if walking on needles*. It selects particularly joints with synovial capsules such as the knee but also has a particular affinity for the deltoid muscle so another modality is *< lifting anything*. Characteristically they cannot grasp things such as cups. The itch comes through on the mental level as *irritability*. They are the archetypal crotchety old colonel. *Rhus toxicodendron* also has an affinity for the long bones so comes up as a remedy for growing pains (a form of rheumatism) especially of the thighs. Another characteristic is the sweat. They will sweat profusely with rheumatics (!) especially at night and the acute symptoms come on after unaccustomed or over-exertion win which the sweat has been checked by too rapid cooling down.

> **EXERCISE**
>
> Create a table of comparison between *Rhus toxicodendron, Rhododendron, Rumex crispus, Ranunculus bulbosa, Ruta graveolus* and *Arnica*.

Remedy	Rhus tox	Rhod	Rumex	Ranunculus	Ruta	Arnica
Exciting Cause						
Affinity						
Sensation						
Keynotes						
Modalities						

Apis mellifica We use this remedy where there is excess oedema with rheumatism. It comes into three situations. Firstly, it affects synovial capsules such as in the knee where there is much swelling due to fluid. It is especially worse on the *right side*. The knee is very large, *shiny with a rosy glow* and the skin *pits easily on pressure* retaining the pit for some time. Careful though because there is a *great sensitivity to touch* or pressure! The pain *burns and stings* and is much *worse for heat* of any kind. When single joints are affected like this, *Apis* occurs as an acute of constitutional remedies such as *Calcarea* or *Natrum Sulphuricum*. The irritable, flightiness of *Apis* may be present. The symptoms are more likely to be local, starting with *restlessness* of the parts affected then extending to mental restlessness as the disease deepens. *Apis* comes in as an acute of the chronic in many rheumatic situations where the pathology is advanced and there is a problem in uptake of fluid by the capillaries. This may or may not come with kidney dysfunction and may have the complication of High Blood Pressure. What we now see is the end game of oedema collecting in the extremities. As the disease further advances the lungs may become affected by fluid causing *breathlessness*. The patient is intolerant to heat and extremely irritable. When you are thinking of other remedies like *Rhus tox.*, the shininess and the pitting oedema will point you to *Apis*. The third situation to be considered is Rheumatoid Arthritis when there is much swelling and burning pain. The auto-immune response here is akin to the reactivity of the *Apis*.

> **EXERCISE**
>
> Create a table of comparison between *Apis mellifica*, *Arsenicum* and *Rhus toxicodendron*.

Remedy	Apis mellifica	Rhus tox	Arsenicum
Exciting Cause			
Affinity			
Sensation			
Keynotes			
Modalities			

Ledum palustre affects the lower extremities insidiously creeping upwards as chill and purple coloration. Affected parts are chilly even to touch The circulation is poor. Traditionally this is a remedy said to be brought on by over-indulgence, especially to alcohol. This patient is often quite *run down*. Parts are congested so the soles are tender and painful to walk on. This remedy is worse on the *left side* but the problem soon extends to the right. Where the system fails to detox, the skin is affected, looking blotchy an generally unhealthy, and crystals of uric acid build up in the joints creating inflammation. The big toe swells, is hot with throbbing pain << heat. The patient is generally chilly and grumpy.

> **EXERCISE**
>
> Create a table of comparison between *Ledum, Arnica, Lycopodium* and *Lachesis*.

Remedy	*Ledum*	*Arnica*	*Lycopodium*	*Lachesis*
Exciting Cause				
Affinity				
Sensation				
Keynotes				
Modalities				

A Diet for Arthritis

Like all diets, finding a diet for arthritis is individual and medical advice should be sought where great change is undertaken. Do not go in for extremes. The general principle is to feed the body good quality food and promote elimination. Thus, 'junk' food should be avoided. This can generally be defined as over-processed food or food to which preservatives have been added in whatever form, chemical or as fat, sugar and salt. Much modern food tends to be unnaturally over-acid by the addition of salt, sugar and fats. Good food preparation should retain the natural elements of the food. This does not mean you have to eat everything raw. Indeed the Chinese will tell us that some constitutions are too cold to take cold foods and this applies to many arthritics. Yet other foods will overheat the body unnaturally causing irritation – the *Solanacaea* have already been mentioned. Basically, you want to find a diet that suits you and promotes your optimum health. Here are some thoughts for you to consider in finding the best diet for you.

BREAKFAST is the most important meal of the day. Do not kid yourself that you cannot stomach breakfast. If we are setting up a more natural rhythm for the body look at your overall pattern as to when and what you eat. The liver does its detoxifying work overnight during the fast period. Do you allow your body its necessary daily fast? In our society, food is very much a social event so we tend to eat in the evening when the body does not need fuel. Indeed, it needs to fast. You need to compromise here, but:

Rule 1   Do not eat after 6pm (or take a light easily digested snack).

You will do your day's work on your breakfast so make it appropriate. Remember the old adage: breakfast like a king, lunch like a prince and dine like a pauper.

The best breakfast for creating alkalinity is oatmeal porridge. If like me, you do not like it, you could take wheat-free, sugar-free oatcakes. The milk will give you protein and honey will add some of nature's goodness. Dairy-free? You could use rice milk or soya milk or add apple juice or another appropriate fruit juice [1] to wet it. Or you could use a good muesli. These come in so many varieties I am sure you will find one to your taste.

Now you have the basic sustenance that also includes enough daily roughage you can add the vitamins and minerals in the form of nuts and seeds and fruit. The nuts and seeds may provide the protein if you miss out milk. Fruit may be a breakfast on its own stewed or raw. You can add molasses or honey or even yoghurt.

I encourage my patients to see diet as an adventure into a new world or even an indulgence in tastes, but also do not give diets that are elaborate, complicated or confusing. In dire cases even adding an apple or a little good quality honey can vastly improve the quality of food eaten at breakfast.

Still craving your toast? OK but avoid sugary spreads. Use molasses, black treacle or honey or one of the comfitures of fruit without sugar added.

Beverages   Start the day with a glass of water, preferably hot, to get the kidneys flowing. Then keep stimulating drinks to a minimum. Use fruit or vegetable juices – watch the salt and tomato content of proprietary brands of the last. Fruit and herb teas come in many varieties. Today juicers are easily available. I have a patient who starts the day with juiced watercress, celery, carrot and ginger. This is full of goodness for arthritics and cools the body of the rheumatic. *Experiment and indulge. Look after yourself.* If you have to take tea, try green tea which clears mucus – a sign of over-acidity.

Fruits   that are less acid include apples, pears, grapes, bananas, apricots, dates, figs, avocado. Bananas contain a lot of potassium, avocados are a rich source of protein. When not in season you can take them dried. They taste lovely steeped overnight in a little water and honey!

Rule 2   Avoid acid forming foods such as sugar, salt, citrus fruits and dairy produce.

---

[1] Fruit juice is just that, the juice extracted from fruit with perhaps some water to dilute – nothing else. It is not squash or any other concoction that is today called juice by some of my patients.

LUNCH is best enjoyed with friends! This is where we can get into wonderful salads and delicious soups. Do not think that salad is just lettuce, tomato and cucumber. *Indulge.*

Salads Carrot, celery, watercress, beetroot, shredded cabbage green or red, spring onions, radishes and lettuce, cucumber but no tomato or peppers will give you lots to choose from. Use rice or cous cous as a staple ingredient. One of my favourite rice salads contains peas, maize corn, apple and onion sometimes with yoghurt, at other times with lemon juice and olive oil. And need I say that the fresher these ingredients then the more vitamins they contain. For especial goodness use sprouted seeds that are full of new life. Sprouted seeds and a bit of Lambs lettuce are things easily grown in pots in your kitchen, or just outside your kitchen door, and one of the richest sources of goodness you will find as a weed in your garden in the form of dandelion leaves. This herb stimulates digestion and the kidneys. You will go a long way to find anything more nutritious and health promoting.

Oils The body needs essential fatty acids as the building blocks of many hormones. You will find these naturally in many seeds and nuts. When pressed these produce a variety of oils that you can add to salads or cook in. Chinese cookery frequently uses sesame oil. Sesame seeds are the richest source of calcium. Sunflower oil is commonly available. You could also try walnut oil and, of course, many nutritionists now strongly recommend olive oil. I like butter, especially unsalted! Flaxseed oil and cod liver oil are frequently recommended as dietary additives for arthritic constitutions, the latter because it contains vitamin D. The most important thing about oils is that they go rancid and are then most unhealthy. Simon Weil in his book, see below, starts his eight weeks by getting you to clear your fridge of old oils.

Rule 3   Your body needs essential fatty acids and vitamins.

Soups How can you beat a pot of soup? For the rheumatic the most important ingredient is celery. The Naturopath will leave out the potato for the arthritic – as well as being a Solanacaea, potato is seen by the Naturopath as leaching potassium from the body making it more acid. Hence why I have not included baked potato in the Lunch menu but do not forget that this could be your treat on special occasions! In moderation is my other recommendation to patients. Soups enable us to bring in vegetables that are not wise eaten raw, especially the onion family such as onions, leeks and garlic – these tackle that excess mucus again and create internal heat. For proteins, we can add lentils and other pulses. One of the most important group of deacidifying vegetables is the Brassicas and these are easily made into soups: cabbage, broccoli, cauliflower, brussels sprouts. My favourite in this last group is kale. Too strong tasting for some, it is full of iron. That other vegetable full of iron, spinach, is also full of oxalic acid, a no-no for this type of constitution. And to really indulge, you can experiment with herbs and condiments to taste. Some excellent herbs for rheumatism are sage and basil. Try also ginger, artichoke and horse radish. Cinnamon is useful for those with a diabetic tendency. Parsley contains iron.

Rule 4   Eat food as fresh as possible so it contains its vitality.

DINNER Do you have any room left? You could do worse than repeat the lunch menu. Traditionally dinner is meat and two veg. The arthritic is usually advised against red meat. In general, many diets will not recommend eating protein after 4pm. You may need to look at your life style and body needs. If you are at work during the day, this may be the only meal you can cook. Now may be the time to enjoy your Brassicas with some easily digestible fish or eggs. Now may be the time for your sweet indulgence. The body coverts carbohydrates into glucose for use in the body but some sugars will raise blood sugar very fast then leave a craving or hunger. *Slow release carbohydrates* are foods such as starches that will keep feeding the body hours after they were eaten.

Rule 5   Avoid extremes. All in moderation.

> **DIET**
>
> What happens when you eat certain foods?
>
> 1. Try a diet of *Solanacaea* and citrus fruits for a week. If you did this as a class you could identify proneness to rheumatic factors above, create a base line then see how different members of the class respond, i.e. how quickly and with what symptoms.
>
> 2. How does abstaining from dairy products affect your proneness to develop rheumatic factors?
>
> 3. Does giving up wheat products make a difference?
>
> Remember you have to abstain long enough to see the effect clearly. I would suggest 2 - 3 weeks, if not longer.

Exercise

This rule here should be not to indulge. Rheumatism and Arthritis is a disease that expresses in the moving parts, of muscles and bone primarily, so how we use these parts can aid or hinder the disease. Overuse of any part needs to be questioned. Movement is part of our life as animals so movement should be part of daily life. Exercise should be part of our lifestyle. Thus the most common exercise for the long bones is walking.

It should be remembered that keeping these bones functioning at their optimum also enhances the immune system since it is these that produce red blood cells in the bone marrow. Also, it is the muscles of the legs that pump blood back up through the abdomen thus stimulating the abdominal organs and preventing congestion and constipation! Sedentary types traditionally suffer the ills of constipation. A 'constitutional' before a meal is an excellent idea.

I have already mentioned the virtues of Yoga, Tai Chi and Qi Gong remedially. There are three basic Qi Gong exercises, the Deer, the Crane and the Turtle but, since these differ for males and females, I am going to suggest you find a good teacher. To help you on your way I am going to include below just a few that I teach to my patients. The most important principle is not to strain or overdo it. **Little and often** is the key here.

The next most important principle is **breathing** and this is why I particularly like Qi Gong and am pleased to see its availability increase. Next, at whatever level, the exercises should include **stretch and internal massage**. At whatever level, be as gentle and slow as you need to and do only as much or **go as far as you feel comfortable.** You should never feel sore or exhausted after exercise. It is a natural function of the body.

STRESS BUSTER FOR THE SPINE AND UPPER TORSO

These three exercises come from Kum Nye, a Tibetan Yoga system. They are meditative exercises so you need to relax the body and slow down the mind to get the best out of them. You do them as slowly as possible, that is very very slowly. I give them below merely as physical exercises but be aware that they are much more than that. *Further resource Kum Nye.*

1. Gently and slowly roll the neck forward, to the left, back then to the right three times then repeat to the other side. Rest.

2. Sitting in a relaxed position with the spine erect and your hands resting in your lap slowly raise the shoulders up around your ears. When high enough bring your head down between your shoulders to meet them. Then just as slowly and gently raise your head back to its position and lower your shoulders. Do three times. Rest.

3. Sitting with your spine erect and your hands resting in your lap, slowly turn your shoulders or upper pectoral axis of the spine to the right then back slowly before repeating to the left slowly. Keep your eyes pinned to a point in front and do not move the head!

If I say that each of these turns may take five minutes, you may be aware that this system of exercise is so deep it connects to the emotions. Stop and rest at any point. Ideally, you are working with intent rather than will and that is an important point for the arthritic because arthritis is often an emotional problem or attitude that intrudes the will into the body where it does not belong.

The next two exercises I have taken from the *Complete System of Self-Healing* by Dr. Stephen Chang. They emphasis other aspects of the Rheumatic/Arthritis constitution.

THYROID MASSAGE

This can be effectively done with the Plough exercise in Hatha Yoga but once the degenerative state has set in, that could be a little dangerous to perform! The thyroid is found in the throat area so simply apply pressure and stimulate movement on your throat on either side of the windpipe. As the thyroid controls the rate of metabolism and the arthritic's metabolism is often slow as well as congested, this stimulates the body to eliminate toxins more effectively.

BONE BREATHING

I love this exercise and even teach it to the crippled osteoporosis patient. Dr. Chang states:
"Taoists have understood for centuries that the best way to protect against disease is to give oneself a full body and mind relaxation at least once a day. Relaxation is of the utmost importance for healing to take place, as it helps prevent energy blocks caused by the build up of tension."

To do the exercise lie comfortably on your back with your legs slightly apart and your hands by your side with the palms turned upwards. Relax with eyes closed and breathe normally. Then, as you inhale, feel the air enter into and penetrate your body bringing clean fresh air, energy and vitality. As you exhale do not just visualise but feel the toxins leave your body. *(Connecting to real body feeling undoes the will in the body.)*

Now, when you inhale, concentrate on feeling the air enter through your toes, flowing up through the bones in your leg and into your chest. Then feel it descend again as you breathe out. Take time to do this 2-3 times with each leg then move on and feel the air come in through your hand, up your arm to your chest. Repeat with each hand. Remember to relax deeply and give yourself up to the healing powers of the air which is the breath of life.

EIGHT STRANDS OF THE BROCADE

It is said that these exercises were practised by the Emperors of China. They are the most effective I know for tonifying and healing the sagging, congested internal organs of the devitalised. I was taught them by a healthy young Vietnamese monk who did them very fast as in Kung Fu! Other monks I have seen do them at a more sedate pace. Their idea is to do them with mindfulness. The Vietnamese monk concentrated on the breath shooting out through the outstretched part. Do them at a pace you feel comfortable with, feeling your body sigh with pleasure as the energy flows into tired parts. Traditionally each is done eight times. When I am fit and do them faster I can do more than that or less if I have been sitting for weeks stressed and congested. The exercises are done in order.

1. Stand with your legs a little apart (or sit if your are really devitalised). The knees should be loose and not tense. Raise your arms so your hands are resting palms up on top of your head. Now, as you stretch your arms up, palms together, breathe out then in as you lower them back to rest on your head. This exercise is said to stimulate.

2. In the same standing position, draw a bow across your chest, i.e. as one arm draws back at shoulder height the other shoots straight out to the side like an arrow as you breathe out. Then, as you pull the outstretched arm back to shoulder height, shoot out the other breathing out. Of course, you can only breathe out again if you have breathed in whilst changing arms.

3. Still in standing position, push one arm up straight and vertical with the palm facing upwards at the same time as the other arm pushes down to the ground with the palm facing down. Then reverse the arms. Breathe out with the stretch.

4. Next, still in standing position, in front of your solar plexus, hold one hand above the other, palms facing as if you are holding a ball between them, i.e. they should be about a foot apart. Turn the top half of your body to one side and push the palms outward and upwards away from you as if deflecting a blow. Or if you raise your eyes in the same direction this exercise is called *cow gazing at the moon*. Bring your hands back to the ball position as you breathe in before turning and repeating the exercise to the other side.

5. In standing position, bring one arm up curving over your head as the other weighs down to the ground down. Your heel is also raised as you stretch one side of your body. Relax and let your arms exchange places so you can stretch the other side.

6. You get to move your legs a little further apart in this one. Start with your arms outstretched before you. Keep your head up facing forwards but bend over as you pull the arms in a downward curve backwards. Do you remember as a child you played at horses? The movement is here more exaggerated. This exercise stimulates kidney energy.

7. Back to the standing position as you form a fist and pull the bow forwards stretching out one arm as you pull the other back into the shoulder, then reverse the arms. This one looks very like a common karate poise.

8. In the last exercise stand with the feet together and the hands pressed into the kidney area at the back. Breathe in, in, in and then further in then out, out, out and further out as you allow the body to shake out all its tension. An invigorating one to finish with.

Now rest.

Different teachers teach these exercises with different emphasis. When I was originally taught Tai Chi by a Chinese Master he encouraged us to make it our own and to tune into the body's energy moving slowly and sensing the breath. Find yourself a teacher.

> **EXERCISE**
>
> How much exercise is enough? Well, how much do you do?
>
> 1. Keep a weekly diary of the type and amount of exercise you do in a typical week.
>
> 2. What is the ideal for your constitution? Change your plan, experiment and see how that affects you over the long and short term.
>
> 3. It would be ideal to compare this with your classmates or family members of different ages, and constitutional types.

Remedies

Natrum muriaticum

This is not a remedy you will find in your First Aid box as it is a constitutional remedy of such deep maladies as cancer, Crohn's disease, multiple sclerosis, psoriasis, clinical depression and rheumatoid arthritis. I put it in this section to show you the scope of a homoeopathic remedy and to give you some idea of the machinations and complexities of disease viewed homoeopathically. For instance, one arthritis type is the acerbic old dame whose grief or disappointed love has turned her into a resentful recluse who keeps her feelings to herself so as not to be hurt again. You will often see suppressed strong emotions behind arthritic cases. The disease is a general withdrawal of the life forces from the deepest parts of the skeleton. The loss of love, or to feel *abandoned and unlovable,* is the most lifeless of all loves.

Natrum muriaticum is Latin for sodium chloride, common salt. In all organism life, it influences the osmotic pressure between cells so enabling each cell to absorb nutrients and exchange waste products. Yet, think what happens when you eat too much salt. You get thirsty, the mucus membrane of the mouth dries. The parched lips become hard as well as dry. Many of the eruptions of *Natrum muriaticum* are herpetic – they start dry then crack and weep as the skin is over tight. The theme runs through the remedy so the stool is often very hard at the start then, when the 'plug' passes, the stool is even loose, *Natrum muriaticum* is a remedy of opposites.

It is very closely related to water (the salinity of the oceans causes the movement of ocean currents) which is a polar compound. Osmotic pressure relies on two 'opposites', two liquids of different degree of concentration, so the water is pulled through to the stronger solution until equilibrium is established. Yet, the essence of *Natrum muriaticum* is more than this because it forms a hard barrier to stop exchange. This is the crust of the eruption, the hard plug of the stool, and the rigid barrier to feeling that prevents further hurt.

They are vulnerable, deeply sympathetic types, one of the few truly altruistic people, who come across as very hard and calculating. They have indeed measured what is required of them, sometimes because they have been cut off at such a young age by grief that they do not know what is appropriate so have learned rationally rather than through relationships. They have no spontaneity. They clunk along the corridor with purpose. Were you to ask them how they walk, i.e. to think about it, they cease up and cannot put one foot in front of the other. In later stages, or as in multiple sclerosis, transmission along the nerves is interrupted and they become clumsy. It is part of their premenstrual syndrome.

Their speech may be staccato, or at best short blunt sentences. They are frank, rational people who call a spade a spade and may have little expertise in small talk. Their dress is often plain and lifestyle correct and without frills. Correctness may lead them into many campaigns for good causes or lead them to a concern for health. They are often carers or in the health professions, or teachers. Their motivation may well be that others will not suffer as they have done. Their honesty may make them very difficult to live with. They are not flatterers so do not ask their opinions if your do not want it! Living by logic and rationality, they may want to sit down and talk a lot about how things are in a relationship. It may be a bit strident to some.

Thus, their nerves often suffer. They can be over-tense. Ardent *time keepers* they are often late because they have measured that there will be time to do one more thing. They are overburdened with things to do because they care so much yet do it all so thoroughly they become over-stressed. They will push themselves to a nervous breakdown with their exacting schedules, or the organism breaks down. They suffer migraine headaches with *visual disturbances of zig zags*. The headache is noticeably < rest times such as weekends or holidays, i.e. *when they relax* and let their guard down. The headache also points to another keynotes. They are *worse around 10am*. The headache *starts at 10am then* gets worse with the sun and improves towards evening. They are < *sun* and < *sunrise to sunset*. It is one of the remedies of prickly heat. They are also < *seaside* where there are higher levels of salt in the air. They are < *in the morning on rising*. This especially applied to the depressive who cannot face the day ahead when they think of it but is well as soon as they are up and at it, > *occupied*. They need to be in relationship and loved but alas avoid this to protect their vulnerability.

Their frequent colds may start as a watery discharge that excoriates the parts. They may get cold sores when they are below par; or over-anxiety and perfectionism may lead to psoriasis. You will have to question them carefully because, on the one hand, they have their own ideas about health and its causes that you will find very difficult to get around, and on the other hand, they will not admit their feelings or weaknesses. If they have been to 'therapy' they may admit to weaknesses but this will be packaged as 'something they can now cope with, or have dealt with' so they will not talk about it. You need to observe the cold sores and experience the abruptness and over-rationality. It does not appear as a remedy in many other respiratory disorders until we find it in ME that has often been brought on by flu. The symptom is then great debility.

The digestive system easily manifests the disturbance in the *Natrum muriaticum* patient. This is lined with mucus membrane whose very role is exchange. The most common symptoms, especially after over-indulgence in salt, is swollen and engorged mucus membrane that cannot absorb so there is a loose stool and the keynote > *fasting*.

There is another keynote symptom that you will see in cancer and Crohn's disease, *they emaciate whilst eating well*. It is one remedy in particular that benefits from the fad for a wheat-free diet, as they are < bread. Alas, they crave salt. They have sudden attacks of nausea accompanied by sinking strength. The mental picture comes through even here when they do not want to show illness in front of others. Indeed, there is the symptom *cannot pass water in front of the nurse*. They hide their weaknesses and are < *consolation*.

As a hormonal remedy, it affects the period. In particular there is sinking of spirits before menses but there can also be mood swings when they can be hysterical or taciturn at the least slight, or supposed slight. Fertility may be affected when only one ovary releases an egg. This may be indicated first by the PMS affecting only every second period! It can easily cure infertility when that is caused by failure to release the egg. It also helps the woman who finds intercourse too intimate and cannot give herself up to the spontaneity of the hormones.

At menopause, this holding back is seen as dryness in the vagina. Have you seen those old ladies with puckered lips? It is said to correspond to the shrivelled-up womb! In Chinese medicine the womb is related to the heart both as an organ and regards feelings of compassion. They do not even demonstrate their good feelings. At menopause, palpitations accompany the dryness. The rhythm of the heart may also be affected as they skip beats, usually every eleventh it is said. Whilst I have come across *Natrum muriaticum* patients skipping a beat it was not as regular as that. The abruptness is apparent in the suddenness of the heart attack. This abruptness is also seen when they leave a room or a conversation abruptly, sometimes thinking they will not be noticed, despite the thunderous silence.

> **PRACTICE POINT**
>
> If you are in a class where you can be supervised, a proving of *Rhus toxicodendron* might give you deeper understanding of the Rheumatic Factor then anything you can read in a textbook.

READINGS

Simon Weil   Eight Weeks to Optimum Health

A Naturopath applies the wisdom of the ages to modern day life style.

Patrick Holryd   Optimum Nutrition

This book contains a lot of modern research and many questions to aid an exploration of diet.

THOUGHT TO PONDER

Diet must be the basis of all medical therapy, yet diet should not be a treatment in itself.

Paracelsus

LESSON 10 Different Types of Acute Disease

Aims: To understand the role of acute disease.
To identify different types of acute disease.
To evaluate different types of acute disease in terms of energy levels of the Vital Force.
To evaluate different types of acute disease in relation to types of chronic disease.
To evaluate different types of acute disease in terms of potency used.

Key words used:
Total Symptom Picture
One disease
Vital Force
exciting cause
predisposition
resonance
susceptibility
vitality
affinity
maintaining cause
points of change
elimination
disease process
latency

Homoeopathy is probably one of the best known and most used of all alternative medicines. Used with accuracy its curative action is unsurpassed. Why then is there still so much doubt surrounding its efficacy? Alas, I would contend that its remedies are often used without the application of homoeopathic principles especially in regards to encompassing the **Total Symptom Picture**. Do I need to repeat that the Homoeopath treats the totality of expression of the Vital Force, that each case all the symptoms must be understood in the context of the whole? I was much heartened to see that the most recent edition of a well-known medical textbook not only emphasised homoeostasis but ended each section by looking at that system in the context of the whole. The Total Symptom Picture is central to any prescription based on homoeopathic principles.

The Homoeopath sees only **one disease**, i.e. a disturbance of the **Vital Force**, that invisible life energy that holds our blue print and acts ceaselessly each second to correct and hold the integral pattern of who we are, as humans and as individuals. To the Homoeopath, symptoms are not the disease but the evidence that the Vital Force is correcting a disturbance. As long as there are symptoms, there is cure possible but we must work with the symptoms, along the line of their expression, to remove the disturbance to the action of the Vital Force. Thus, we must learn to evaluate the symptoms. Throughout this text, we have been working with symptoms, learning names and values. In this lesson, I want to put it all together to understand the role of the acute. The philosophy is complex so this lesson is mainly for the practitioner. Nevertheless I have added footnotes for the interested patient.

A Simple Acute

Up to Paragraph 71 of his *Organon*, Hahnemann keeps the principles very simple. I have reflected his work up to this point in my text *The Principles of Homoeopathic Philosophy*. Hahnemann himself realised it was a bit more complicated than this when he discovered *'chronic disease'* and we will come to that in a bit.[1]

A simple acute arises from the interaction of an **exciting cause** and the **predispositions**[2] of the Vital Force. The degree of disturbance, or interaction, is determined by the degree of **resonance** (i.e. the susceptibility[3]), by the virility of the exciting cause and by the **vitality** of the person.

---

[1] Or you will find a more detailed study in my other book *Constitutional Prescribing*.

[2] A predisposition is a tendency to act in a certain manner, to reproduce a specific pattern of symptoms because of the affinities, characteristic essence and susceptibility, where the essence is the mode of action of the Vital Force and the susceptibility is the resonance or capability of action.

[3] I have noted a little trouble in my students of late in differentiating homoeopathic susceptibility from the allopathic term. This is unfortunate as susceptibility is one of the most important concepts in Homoeopathy. In more usual Western medicine, susceptibility means prone to because of weakness. In Homoeopathy, it means that to which the Vital Force resonates. Such resonance is usually created by the miasm underlying.

Thus, lowered vitality can make us more prone to 'catch' something [4]. The predisposition explains how we each have our own reaction pattern so some stimuli will not affect us. The exciting cause is the other side of the coin of susceptibility – the lowered vitality is not enough, there has to be stimulation. For example, whilst many may react to tobacco smoke or perfume, to some it acts as a very powerful trigger that may create much distress. The reaction to an exciting cause is not necessarily along the lines of the chemical action of tobacco which is the response to the maintaining cause. Indeed, the individual may produce the same acute pattern with several different exciting causes – it is the drain or channel of least resistance to the flow of symptoms outwards used by the Vital Force in recreating balance. Hence, in one it may produce a runny nose or eyes, in another nausea whilst in another a sore throat or headache. The symptoms produced may show the **affinity**, also **location**, **modality** and **intensity** or degree of disturbance.

Thus, simple acute disease can be recognised by several factors:

1. There is a clear exciting cause.

2. Symptoms are produced relatively quickly – within minutes, hours, seldom a few days.

3. Resolution is equally fast – minutes, hours or a few days.

4. There are no complications – deepening of symptoms into other anatomical systems.

5. There are no symptoms dragging on after the main symptoms have been resolved – the patient either dies or recovers completely.

6. Irrespective of the cause, each person is affected in their 'usual' manner. The affinity represents how the predisposition is activated often irrespective of the trigger or exciting cause, e.g. you are always taking sore throat whilst I take headaches.

VITALITY

There are no complications to a simple acute. The patient either recovers or dies *depending on the intensity of the disturbance.*

Where the vitality is lowered, there is a longer period before the symptoms appear. This indicates *less vitality* with which to respond. We are used to looking at disease as an attack on the organism. This does not fit into a homoeopathic perspective. **Symptoms demonstrate the ability to maintain the integrity of the whole.** It is not disease that is important but health. A healthy Vital Life Force will adapt; the healthier, the faster it will adapt to unhealthy conditions. When looking at a case, the Homoeopath wants to know how quickly it is reacting and, if slow, what stops rapid resolution to the disturbance. The most common cause of lowered vitality of the last is the maintaining cause. When an advanced level of the disease process is common then the lowered vitality may be caused by the miasm.

The **maintaining cause** affects vitality by overburdening the detoxifying processes. This may slow down the ability of the Vital Force to resolve the disturbance. I wrote earlier, in *Principles of Homoeopathy,* that there are five pillars of health – clean air, clean water, clean food, sleep and exercise. Now I would add freedom from stress as represented by noise, haste, doing too much, over-stimulation of nerves in general and emotions in particular.

Vitality is indicated by:

- how fast the symptoms are produced after the Exciting Cause
- the type of Miasm
- the level of disease process expressed at that point.

Acutes are not caused by maintaining causes (even though symptoms might be so caused).

---

[4] To labour such an important point again, proneness is weakened vitality, allowing reaction to a lower threshold of stimuli; susceptibility is that to which the Vital Force is resonance, i.e. interacts with rather than is acted upon.

SUSCEPTIBILITY

Susceptibility is the most important concept in Homoeopathy. To understand this is to understand the homeopathic perspective on disease. It is subtly different from an allopathic understanding of susceptibility. The Allopath will talk of susceptibility as a weakness. It is much more than that to a Homoeopath.

The Vital Force is not a passive object to be acted upon. Nothing penetrates an energy field but that to which it is resonant. OK a delicate one might be disrupted by a blast of crude energy, but the colour red is not affected by anything other than light or another energy form in a resonant octave. The Vital Force is not acted upon but interacts. This subtle difference is expressed in a case at the **points of change**, those points at which the pattern of symptoms changes. The **exciting cause** is the major factor here.

In the simple acute, the exciting cause throws the Vital Force off balance. The Vital Force then throws out symptoms to recover balance, like the ripples spreading out on a pond surface when we drop in a stone.

In a complex chronic case, over a life time, there may be several points at which the symptom picture has changed, usually deepened, i.e. to express disturbance in more complex anatomical systems. The reasons are complex but hinge around increased or decreased vitality. To find a remedy that resonates at these points is to engage the Vital Force and *susceptibility* but now we are in the realms of chronic disease, the miasm – see below.

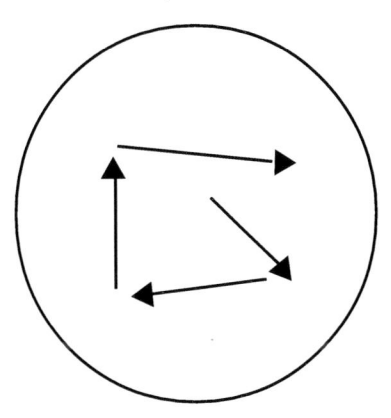

When a homoeopathic remedy engages these points there is an increase in the energy of the Vital Force with a corresponding increase in symptoms or in the movement of symptoms. This is because these are points where healing has not been completed because of lowered vitality, the miasm or blocking maintaining causes. With more energy, the flow starts again. The wise Homoeopath, knowing the Vital Force has been engaged, treads warily, usually watches and waits. This is no longer a simple acute.

The Psoric Acute

This is really the simple acute but I have given it a different name because I want to emphasise different properties of the Vital Force. **The Vital Force does not need an outside trigger to produce the acute. It will do so when vitality rises.** To understand this we need to know the role of the acute in relation to chronic disease.

First, an acute is a group of symptoms that represents the resolution of disturbance. As disturbance is resolved, energy is freed up so **the acute increases the vitality of the person.** Likewise, as the person increases in vitality, they may have the energy to produce an acute that will change the level of expression, or predisposition – although more usually it is only the level of the disease process that is changed. This is represented in some Psoric remedies, especially *Psorinum,* when they are so well before they are ill!

More often, this type of acute will arise after homoeopathic treatment as the remedy increases the vitality. The Vital Force will use the acute expression of disease to further correct disturbance or imbalance on the level of chronic disease, and so further create more energy and better health. We could call this a detoxification process. In psoric terms, it is an **elimination.**

A change in the level of health is not possible to the Homoeopath without the movement outwards of the symptoms, which happens in an acute.

This accounts for the phenomenon after homoeopathic treatment when the patient has one more attack whether it be the clean out diarrhoea of food poisoning or an asthmatic attack or epileptic fit. You need a bit of knowledge and experience before you attempt homoeopathic constitutional treatment! It is for this reason also that the Homoeopath dislikes patients exciting the Vital Force with the use of randomly prescribed homoeopathic remedies. Were they to engage the Vital Force ... Fortunately, you have to be very accurate with homoeopathic remedies to awaken the sleeping dragon of the miasm.

The Acute Miasm

Why are Homoeopaths disturbed when a case shows no occurrence of childhood diseases? We inherit the genetic material of our parents with a constitutional pattern already imprinted. The doctor will not argue with that but the Homoeopath will go further in saying that this is also a debilitated level of energy with an imprinted pattern of chronic disease, a miasm. However, usually the child has more energy than the adult so will attempt to correct the imbalance by producing an acute illness. The Homoeopath has observed that these are related to the underlying type of constitution inherited [5] and further, after the acute childhood illness, the presentation of symptoms changes levels indicating an improvement in vitality. Put plainly, the role of the acute childhood illness to the Homoeopath is to clear out the inherited dross and use the energy of childhood to create a better level of health.

The childhood illnesses [6] are thus called acute miasms because they express and change the ultimate level of expression of the inherited miasm, or chronic disease. Each childhood disease is linked to a specific miasm, hence in today's world:

Psora	links to	Measles
Sycosis		Mumps
Syphilis		Chicken-pox
Tubercular		Croup/Whooping cough
Cancer		Whooping cough

Historically, the first four are milder forms of *Scarlet fever, Smallpox, Polio,* and *Diphtheria* respectively. The history of the development of diseases is a fascinating topic. Now we are not speaking the same language as the doctor and, whilst arousing your interest, I am going to keep this door closed until there is much more discussion of *chronic disease*.

Suffice it to say that the acute miasm follows the form of the Psoric acute. It arises generally when there is increased health to deal with it. It resolves of its own accord usually without any complications or continuing consequences. Where we have seen the latter two factors more in evidence recently is where there is much more to clear out than the individual Vital Force is capable of – the miasmic load is increasing because acute disease is suppressed, the maintaining cause level of toxins in day-to-day life is increased and disease is not cured but further complicated by modern suppressive drug treatments. Generally, this indicates deeper levels of the disease process and more complicated *chronic disease* in the population as a whole. The next section will continue explanation.

The Constitutional Case and Health

Firstly, we must understand what is meant by 'constitution'. To the Homoeopath, the constitutional case is the Vital Force at rest having achieved whatever balance is possible.[7] Thus, the constitutional case is a pattern of symptoms that represents the unresolved disease state. The factors that created it may be in the past but there are energies maintaining the balance that the remedy must interact with. What is visible as the character of the constitution is its recognisable personality of 'weaknesses' from which we can recognise the inheritable miasm. No homoeopathic treatment is complete without an attempt to raise the level of health further by treating the constitutional case.

---

[5] Not everyone catches an epidemic. Indeed, it is a very serious epidemic indeed if 25% 'catch it'. The Homoeopath would say we 'catch' illnesses according to our underlying predispositions.

[6] In Hahnemann's day, they were not always childhood illnesses. Adults got them too and often more violently. As the gene pool adapted, they became illnesses of childhood. For a real eye opener read *Plague's Progress* by Arno Karlen or *The White Plague* by Rene Dubois.

[7] Read Rene Dubois *Man Adapting*

If we look at any constitutional case, we are aware of different *levels of expression* of symptoms. Apart from the broad spread through Mental and Emotional symptoms, to Generals and Particulars, there is a characteristic acute that expresses the vitality or level of health, e.g. some will produce the acute in the upper respiratory system as a cold whilst others are more likely to produce bronchitis which is a deeper disturbance because it more seriously affects the respiratory system function. Further there is a hierarchy of *systems* affected and each miasm has its own pattern of degeneration. The *nature* of the constitution arises from the miasms inherited, i.e. whether Psoric, Sycotic, Syphillitic, Tuberculoid, Cancer [8]. The nature of the constitution, or *mode* of expression, combined with the level of expression depending on the level of health will give us the **disease process** showing how skilfully the body's defences have achieved compromise.

Chronic disease is the third option of the Vital Force, not just to die if it cannot recover but to compromise.

The compromise, or adaptation, of chronic disease is achieved at the expense of health. A new centre of gravity is sought so that, if the symptoms cannot reach the edge of the pond, they are contained safely. The disturbance is allowed to manifest more deeply, so that instead of the skin eruption at the edge of the pond now there is respiratory disturbance, or digestive disturbance, depending on the type of constitution. There is a movement from the **sensation** level of disease to the **dysfunction** level. In the process there may be a period of latency whilst the new location and system is disturbed in its function. When the disease is internalised, its nature changes so that it slows down. There is now less vitality to respond swiftly with an acute. The acute may take several days to occur after the exciting cause.

Acutes arise when the constitutional balance is disturbed.

In the first instance, what disturbs the constitutional balance is a change in the vitality or an exciting cause.

When the disturbance is internalised, the process of disease is slowed down.

HOW IS VITALITY CHANGED?

Other than the miasm, a maintaining cause is the most common cause of lowered vitality, and conversely removal of this might increase vitality. Changes in habit, particularly diet and exercise, may rapidly change the level of vitality. For example, we are more prone to illness in Winter because the cold and damp 'wear us down'. Similarly some are prone to illness on holiday, or at weekends, when the maintaining cause level is lifted (e.g. occupational stress) and the Vital Force is free to address some imbalance.

The exciting cause is the strongest agent to change vitality as it disturbs the integrating influence of the Vital Force creating a need for adaptation to correct the pattern. The different type of acutes that arise in a constitutional case are related directly to the level of containment, i.e. the level of the **disease process**. In a simple acute, the balance is restored as before because there is no need to change it.

Since to the Homoeopath we are **all** contaminated by inherited miasms, it could be argued that there is no such thing as a simple acute in reality – it is indeed a teaching model that simplifies the complicated actions of the Vital Force. However, since the miasm is an inherited mutation the balance created by the Vital Force is not easily rocked and the Vital Force has reason to tenaciously hold to that balance achieved so the reaction of most 'healthy' types to the acute produced by the exciting cause is to return to previous balance.

THE ROLE AND TYPES OF ACUTES IN THE CONSTITUTION CASE

Hahnemann tells us that once affected miasmically the Vital Force, thrown out of balance, continues to degenerate thus creating the 'ageing process' where age brings us greater dysfunction in more vital processes. The adaptation of the constitution pushes this into old age for most of us but we are aware that if we abuse our constitution illness arises! Most simple acutes at the constitutional level that arise are correcting such abuse and returning us to the point of balance.

---

[8] A better term might be carcinoid as it does not necessarily involve the disease cancer.

The Acute Miasm and what I have called the Psoric acute can change the baseline, by which we mean they can change the predispositions and even alter the miasm. This also happens after homoeopathic constitutional treatment but it requires such energy that it is most commonly found at those points (of change) where the organism's energy naturally rises to encompass growth points – hence also why such acutes are most common in children. They are found commonly at dentition, secondary dentition, puberty, pregnancy. Where only the level of the disease process is changed I have called this **Constitutional Type A: progressive**, because the miasm remains the same.

At points of change where the change is not accomplished fully, because there is not enough vitality, adaptation is arrested or slowed down. Then we will see a deepening of the symptom picture, a shift in the level of disease process expressed. An example could be a disappearance of the early childhood tonsillitis to an adolescent tendency to bronchitis, or the disappearance of childhood eczema and the appearance of asthma. Such points of change often occur in relation to exciting causes such as shock, grief, fright, exam time, change of house or job, etc. I have called this **Constitutional Type B: regressive** [9]. It is the common ageing process that marches on if there is no treatment.

More often, the role of the acute in a constitutional case is to maintain balance rather than to restore health, but as chronic disease was created as a third option to the kill or cure of the simple acute, the ultimate cure of such miasms is again the acute which is why the Vital Force returns to it time and again when it has the energy to do so. Thus the type of acute produced in a constitutional case gives us a great deal of information. It occurs from changes in vitality and depends on vitality but also shows us the level of energy available for cure, and hence the potency we can employ. Different types of constitution miasmically indicate different levels of vitality. Also, within each constitution, as miasm degeneration (ageing) proceeds there are different accommodations at the level of the disease process which fundamentally mean a slower onset, more protracted incidence and longer recovery period. So, let us summarise the types of acute so far mentioned and determine their relationship to the constitutional case:

Type of Acute	In Terms of Vitality	Comments
Simple	Vitality lowered from abuse of constitution, over-use, over-stressed so no resistance to Exciting Cause. Or look for a very strong EC.	Look at Maintaining Cause as well as Exciting Cause. Treatment restores to balance.
Acute Miasm	Vitality rises naturally at growth points.	Seldom needs treatment unless there are complications. Can shift the miasmic balance.
Psoric Acute	Occurs when vitality rises spontaneously.	May resolve spontaneously or treatment may give access to the miasm for treatment.
Constitutional Type A Progressive	At growth points when increased vitality.	Usually clear EC because more reactive than Type B. Treatment enables a shift in the level of the disease process expressed.
Constitutional Type B Regressive	Stress points that decrease vitality.	Important to distinguish from Type A because there is less vitality so a lower potency is used – aim to restore miasmic balance. Conversely if clear and vigorous EC you may need high potencies (e.g. grief) or a deeper level of disease process results and this becomes a point of change to be treated later. Rule of thumb, the faster the reaction produced then the higher the potency.
Acute after Constitutional Treatment	Occurs as vitality rises.	Enables shift in level of disease process expressed and can even shift miasmic balance.

[9] I have used these terms of progressive and regressive so my senior students can link with the work of Prof. Michael Kirkman

> **EXERCISE**
>
> It would be useful for you to come up with examples of each of these.

The Recurrent Acute

Alas this is more common in these days when the miasms are more likely to be Tubercular or Cancer. These are often called pseudo-miasms because they mirror Psora and Sycosis but at deeper stages in the disease process. They have different characteristics in terms of vitality – vitality is lower – but it is more than that. If I say there was great difficulty finding the tuberculosis bacteria because it took 6 weeks to incubate, unlike the more common Streptococcus and Staphylococcus that reproduce dozens of times in 24 hours, then you may be prepared for some of the characteristics of the pseudo-miasms.

The symptoms are not so clear in Individuality. There are fewer keynotes in a case. Susceptibility too is dulled so you will find fewer exciting causes and response more likely due to the modality. There is much less vitality so it takes longer to produce the symptoms and the crisis is not always resolved as clearly. Indeed the acutes recur because they are inadequately resolved.[10] In the repertory, we find the rubric *tendency to take cold* but, depending on the constitutional remedy, there are also recurrent ear problems, swollen glands, laryngitis, headaches or digestive disturbances. It is as if the gramophone needle has struck, **nothing can be resolved or move on**. Often the case is characterised by low grade fevers that are not high enough for the inflammatory defences to kick in. At best, there may be 2 – 3 colds in the winter but as vitality drops further, they may never really finish one before the next starts.

What is happening to the Vital Force? It is low in vitality so there is less energy to resolve disturbance – it cannot move symptoms to the edge of the pond. The disturbance has been contained at a deeper level because there was so much to express that it was life threatening to push out at a level nearer the surface. The violence of the symptoms would have threatened life. This is the only reason that the Vital Force takes symptoms to express at a deeper level. The advantage gained by this action is that the disease process is slowed down; it might enter a stage of **latency** while it constructs another pattern of expression. The recurrent acute comes before this adaptation has been completed, i.e. when the Vital Force is still trying to create a better level of health. What we must always remember in treating chronic disease is that the way back to health is through the level of greater violence in the symptoms. That is why homoeopathic constitutional prescribing should be done only by the trained Homoeopath who can follow the change in remedies and alter potency to handle aggravations, who knows the meaning of the acute presentation.

When we treat the recurrent acute, our objective must be resolution, to bring the Vital Force to a point where it can get over the hump and let go of the old pattern. At first, we may not stop the acutes occurring but, if you study these acutes, now you will see the patient's energy shift after them. The patient will feel better in themselves, they will sleep better, they will have better bowel motions, their appetite will be better, there will be less complications in their menses, i.e. the **General** symptoms improve. They will not feel such malaise. And these acutes will now be more violent, or stronger in their action.

Even greater success will see an interesting homoeopathic phenomenon in which there will be one more and severe incidence of the acute. As the energy rises there is an attempt to resolve the pattern at that level so allowing a shift in the level of the disease process. So, for example, recurrent bronchitis may become simple colds, then merely one cold and only when the exciting cause presents. The aggravation is always in the channels already open, or in related channels of expression according to Hering's Laws of Cure.

---

[10] And alas, you need to distinguish this from acutes that recur repeatedly from modern habits of taking suppression drugs to quell the symptoms such as fever that are the organism's first line of defence.

The potency used varies depending on the vitality and the particular **affinity** of the indicated constitutional remedy. Unless it is really life threatening, we do not use the acute remedy here but the constitutional remedy in a low potency such as the 30th where it can act on the general level. We may increase potency as the acute changes to higher levels of expression, e.g. from the lungs to the tonsils. Where the aggravation is controlled by the acute remedy, you might find even more energy through the cleared drains so more violent symptoms.

Usually when this happens the patient feels great, even though ill! The acute remedy is also appropriate where the resolution is slow and dull, to speed up response through more energy in the system. Alternatively, the acute remedy can be used to slow down the violence by controlling the potency. When you study the case you must look for the drain and channels of expression and ask if there is anything that might 'block' the action of the remedy and thus cause complications, i.e. maintaining causes.

Episodic Acute

You will see this written about in the textbooks. It took me some time to understand it fully. At first glimpse, it is simply an acute that recurs periodically. Many acutes will recur especially if related to an exciting cause that is seasonal for any reason. This is not the same as the above recurrent acute for two reasons: it does not signify lowered vitality, indeed it may be the opposite; it is marked by **periodicity**. When periodicity occurs in a case, you will recognise the higher vitality by clearer, more individualistic symptoms and by clear response to an exciting cause, i.e. a qualitative difference.

If we go back to the three causes of acute disease being a meeting with the exciting cause, lowered vitality and according to the predisposition of the underlying chronic disease then the recurrent acute comes about by lowered vitality whilst the episodic acute is primarily a meeting with the exciting cause, although it could be the **raised vitality** of Spring. Thus, a good example of an episodic acute is Hay Fever, which occurs in the Spring when pollen, the **exciting cause**, arrives on the scene. However, I must point out that many cases of Hay Fever I see today are not episodic acutes even though they recur every Spring; they are more a result of much lowered vitality which we could put down to continued degeneration along miasmic lines, i.e. recurrent acutes that are further depressed by the exciting cause which now acts like a maintaining cause. The remedies required in these last cases are 'sub-acute' in modern terminology, e.g. *Pulsatilla* rather than *Allium cepa* or *Arsenicum*.

Malaria was Hahnemann's example of an episodic acute. Here it is much more difficult to see any relationship to an external factor, even an exciting cause. Malaria recurs yearly in many. It points to the nature of the chronic disease that has a pattern of symptoms that includes periodicity. When we study the old *materia medicas*, there is so much periodicity in remedies. There are clear **Time** aggravations that are individualistic of remedies, that enable differentiation, e.g. *Belladonna* aggravates at 3pm whilst *Apis* which can be so similar aggravates at 4pm. We seem to have lost these clear peaks of the symptom picture in a much more devitalised population.

Indeed, I often find the aggravation of such remedies at the opposite of the clock which puzzled me for years until I realised it was not the acute picture on the **General** level, with clear **exciting cause,** that I was seeing but an acute expressing itself on deeper levels in the system and with clearer **Modalities**. It was not the high fever of *Belladonna* but the sore throat or ear. This is a very different illness needing lower potencies because it has less vitality than the high fever with radiating heat. Back to Malaria, it has the **Time** aggravation of the psoric type case although in others it may arise because of depressed vitality for whatever reason.

When dealing with the episodic acute, for example Hay Fever, you will hear prescription repeated yearly or even that it takes several years to cure. This is because ultimately it is the chronic disease that needs attention, not its acute expression. However, such acute expression is often life threatening when it is asthma or epilepsy so it needs attention to the acute. The episodic acute has the violence of a healthy person. It is not related to the recurrent acute.

Acute of the Chronic

I use this term in relation to great dysfunction of the system so that symptoms are 'chronic' in the orthodox use of that term. The patient has no relief from symptoms and those symptoms cause great debility and distress. An example might be emphysema or osteo-arthritis. There is usually structural change so any effect of the homoeopathic remedy must be slow or cause greater suffering. Thus, Crompton Burnett and J. H. Clarke in their many writings use 2X, 3X, 6X, as well as 6C. Others will talk of organ remedies and 'drainage'.

From this picture of great discomfort, the Vital Force may still attempt to change the level of disease manifestation. When it does so it throws out an acute crisis of elimination – yet this excess exudate gives little relief, indeed usually the opposite, because it is an *'overspill'*. The pains and inflammation of arthritis may be increased savagely after the patient is soaked or after an extra long walk, or shock. The *extra effort* demanded increases the symptoms. Notice that the disease is *well established* and the symptoms represent a *balance* that prevents the disease overcoming the patient. It will overwhelm and cause death when the disorder reaches the major vital organ but for now it is held at arm's length. The main characteristic of such a symptom picture, from the standpoint of homoeopathic philosophy, is that the greater suffering is produced by **Modalities** that become slighter and slighter as the vitality drops further.

Such cases are often heavily medicated – and not just for the symptoms of the illness but also for the side effects of the drugs used so that it may be common to take 10 drugs daily. Such a case needs skilled case management to relieve the **maintaining cause** level and slowly to increase vitality. What you must remember is that the symptoms are the process of cure and therefore may be expected to increase as the remedy increases the Vital Force's ability to cure. In such a situation, we might choose to palliate or use the second best remedy! It is one of the few situations in which we might use repeat doses of the remedy because change will be very slow and may need support, or continual nudging. We use a low potency such as the 6th because there is little energy to work with. Ideally, we will get to a point where we can increase the potency and go back to a single dose! It may take months of carefully monitoring.

Where does epidemic, endemic, sporadic, contagious fit in?

To complete the review of acute prescribing I need to include Hahnemann's categories of acute disease. I have already spoke of these in my *Principles of Homoeopathic Philosophy*. When he uses them, he speaks of the **Simple Acute**. They may also fit into the categories of the **Psoric Acute** and **Constitutional Type A and B** above.

Now we are right into a homoeopathic understanding of disease in terms of the interaction between the exciting cause, vitality and the predisposition. To the Homoeopath there is only **one disease**, a disturbance of the Vital Force's ability to maintain harmony. But, the Vital Force is energetic in nature, 'dynamic' is the word Hahnemann uses, and there it is not acted upon but interacts or resonates. Further, it is very specific regards what it will resonate with and that is determined by its own **nature**, its predispositions which are derived from the warp of the miasm. The predispositions determine the **Susceptibility** or the exciting cause with which it resonates. Vitality lowers or raises the threshold of response. So, each of the four types of acute disease proposed by Hahnemann refer to different relationships of these three factors.

In the **epidemic** acute, the Vital Force responds when predisposition meets its **exciting cause**. Yet, not everyone 'catches' an epidemic. Indeed the actual percentage is very low, usually well below 10%. A recent flu epidemic did not reach epidemic levels because the figures for England and Wales had to be 500/100,000 whilst those for Scotland had to be 1000/100,000 – *because in Scotland they are more liable to flu because of the wet, cold weather*. In percentage figures that is 0.5% and 1% respectively! I first started to study influenza when many cases arising after Haley's comet passed required *Nux vomica*, not a common remedy of flu. That Christmas another wave required *Natrum muriaticum*. I noted that the first group were *out of harmony* and was amazed that these were the same patients that presented with the *Natrum muriaticum* flu but now there was the financial and emotional stress of Christmas. *Natrum muriaticum* is also a remedy that holds on to past conditions. The exciting cause of these remedy types predisposed them to 'catch' this flu. Other examples of epidemics are cholera in hot waterless summers. Who gets the diarrhoea? Who is most likely to succumb? Who gets the cold in the office? As well as their exciting cause, vitality has to be lowered hence the same people in the office do not always catch the cold and the cholera epidemic is more common in war-torn countries in present days, and it is not always due to disruption of water supplies.

In the **endemic** acute, the illness is related to the geographical vicinity where there is a powerful morbific agent such as malaria and swamp fever in swamps, and sleeping sickness where tsetse fly dominate. The last gives an example where the natives' adaptations provide immunity to other illnesses; in this case, sickle cell anaemia gives some immunity to malaria, i.e. the underlying predisposition is changed. Again, not everyone succumbs and it would appear the morbific agent weakens the **vitality** seeping the ability to maintain health, or lowering the threshold.

The **sporadic** acute seeks out those with a greater degree of resonance to the condition, i.e. underlying **predisposition**. This resonance is their exciting cause. It has their name on its destination ticket.

I have spoken elsewhere that **contagion** [11] is not what we would call infectious disease today. Again it is associated with resonance but here it is the underlying **fundamental cause**, or miasm, that predisposes. Into this category would fall the acute miasms that strike according to the underlying miasm. More recent examples might be mass emotional responses, or mass hysteria – grief that has followed death of public figures, outrage or anger at other events. Sport seems to generate more than its fair share of these episodes but more recently crime and politics has moved many people. Why is emotion such an easy example? Perhaps because it is a social experience.

Potency and the Acute

Throughout this text, I have tried to give an idea of potency based on symptoms where symptoms indicate the vitality and speed of action of the Vital Force. The underlying premise is that, as we match the symptoms of the remedy to those of the Vital Force, so we match the energy of the remedy to the energy of the Vital Force. We can use potency to speed up the Vital Force. Indeed the homoeopathic remedy introduces more energy into the system in the sense that it creates greater movement of symptoms. Elements that might influence the choice of potency are therefore:

- Speed of onset of symptoms
- Defence mechanism used by the Vital Force
- Whether the symptoms are at the Sensation, Dysfunction or Structural level
- Whether the Predisposition, Exciting Cause or Vitality predominates as a factor
- Length of duration and change in the symptoms
- The presence of Maintaining Causes
- Type of Miasm involved
- Type of acute involved.

---

[11] In *Constitutional Prescribing*

Lesson 10

READINGS

George Vithoulkas — The Science of Homoeopathy

Well, when you have read this Vithoulkas will provide a thorough approach to homoeopathic philosophy without the complications of the case as above!

Harris Coulter — Modern Medicine and Homoeopathic Science

This will help you talk to the medical profession in its own language.

THOUGHTS TO PONDER

*If two **dissimilar** diseases meet together in the human being and they are either of equal strength, or the **older** one happens to be **stronger**, then the older disease will keep the new one away from the body.*

Someone who is already suffering from a serious chronic disease will not be affected by an autumnal dysentery or other moderate epidemic disease.

From Para 36

*Or the new **dissimilar disease is stronger**. In this case, the weaker disease that the patient already has is postponed and suspended by the stronger supervening disease until the new one has run its course or been cured, and then the old one comes forth again **uncured**.*

From Para 38, The Organon of the Medical Art
Samuel Hahnemann
(Translated by Wendy Brewster O'Reilly)